FOREWORD

No single profession has a monopoly on the treatment or care of the feet. This may explain why there is so little information available about the need for footcare. There has only been one major study on the subject, conducted by a sociologist using chiropodists as assistants. This work is now fourteen years old, and much has changed in the services which provide footcare. This new book has been written by a chiropodist in collaboration with a social scientist, each contributing their own expertise and perspective.

Since 1974, when the previously fragmented services were gathered under the umbrella of the National Health Service, many improvements have been made, although provision is still poor and varies greatly across the United Kingdom.

This book covers the existing problems, and highlights the need for adequate footcare. It is written not only for chiropodists, but for all who can play a part in planning and providing footcare: doctors, nurses, local authorities, voluntary organisations, the shoe trade, health educators, and the Department of Health and Social Security.

It contains not only a description of the research undertaken, but makes concrete proposals for future developments. The reforms suggested are exciting and long overdue, and not all require large injections of finance.

I hope this book is widely read, so that those people who need foot treatment can one day be provided with the care they need.

Donald F. Beaton
District Chiropodist
June 1983

ACKNOWLEDGEMENTS

Our thanks are due to many people who have helped us through the three years of this project. Without the moral and material assistance which have been given so unstintingly, the work would not have been started, much less completed.

In particular, we would like to record our thanks to Don Beaton, then Area Chiropodist of the City and East London Area Health Authority (Teaching), who both found the money and the other resources to sustain the project.

Additionally, other Area staff deserve special mention: Mr M. Malone-Lee, Dr F. Murphy, Mr D. Russell, Dr K. Grant and Mrs J. Sternfield who provided advice and support in their individual ways.

At District level, Dr L. Fry and Mr F. Osborn smoothed access and gave encouragement at all stages. The people in the district to whom we have the greatest debt are those who helped in the field work, especially the chiropodists and their clerical staff, who tolerated a lot of disruption in their routines. We must not forget the school nurses, nor the general practitioners who allowed us access to their work places with such generosity. This was also true of the staff of the Accident and Emergency Department.

The computing was done by the Hill Centre, the London Hospital Medical College; and the typing by Sue Jones and Veronica Roach, who tolerated many changes in the final production of the text.

We would also record our thanks to the Department of Health and Social Security for their help and constructive criticisms.

Last but not least, we owe our thanks to Lady Hamilton and the staff of the Disabled Living Foundation who have made publication possible.

INTRODUCTION

This is the fourth publication about the feet and footwear to be issued by the Disabled Living Foundation (DLF). It is a book the Trustees feel particularly pleased to put forward because of its uniformly constructive approach to problems which are of great importance to a large number of the population, but which have received an almost unbelievable lack of consideration previously.

At the time of writing this foreword the National Health Service is going through a period of difficulty which many of those concerned find disheartening and frustrating. How encouraged DLF feels to publish a report which shows convincingly how a part of the NHS, which concerns such a large proportion of our population, namely the footcare service, can be improved and made available to more patients with substantially the existing staff and no additional costs provided the problems are studied, and the approach reconsidered and modified. Research into the delivery of footcare in relation to need has been so sparse as to be almost non-existent. When it is undertaken, as in this report, the increase in knowledge enables a dramatic reappraisal of the situation from all its aspects.

The research on which the report is based is the work of a highly gifted professional chiropodist, Miss Judith Kemp, and Mr J. T. Winkler, a social scientist, working for one year with practically no funds but assisted by chiropodists and other colleagues in the health district in which the research took place. However, the results of the series of small, well thought out enquiries undertaken, which look for unmet need in the patients and inefficiency in the provision of the service, show that the present strategy for dealing with foot problems will never succeed and that fresh thought and a fresh approach is absolutely imperative.

For example: the failure to give preventive care of children's feet through the school health service results in unmanageable problems at pensionable age. The enquiry found that 90% of school children had a problem either with their shoes or their feet, and that the school nurses (who inspect the children's feet in any event) were not trained for the preventive work which was needed although this could be undertaken (again with no increased expenditure) if the nurses were given some additional briefing. A high proportion of disabled people were found to be in need of chiropody but did not realise that they could get it. Here there is a need for major investigation. The unmet need among the elderly is shown to be enormous. Only those at the tip of the iceberg are receiving needed care largely through routine maintenance which uses up all the professional skill available, and prevents the huge waiting list from obtaining help. There are obviously far too few chiropodists to deal with the vast footcare needs, and this will be so in the foreseeable future no matter what measures are practical to increase their numbers. The only real option is to break out of the impasse by the more efficient use of skills and to fit the spectrum of skills (and there are many of them available) to the spectrum of needs in a better way.

The report recommends many policy changes which have been successfully initiated in the research health district. As national measures, policy changes would cover training of the various disciplines involved, the solution of the problems of the chiropodial profession and of the employment of footcare assistants; the undertaking of much additional research; the improvement of communication between the disciplines involved; and an altogether more vigorous approach to foot health education.

The report is particularly valuable because it deals with so many aspects of the problems of foot health – whether in discussing the need for foot health and fashion to work together (since footwear is the one item of clothing which can damage the body); or in improving the foot health of children (since children's feet do not hurt under deforming footwear and skeletal damage goes on without pain); in discussing the rationing of footcare through the priority group system which clearly does not work, and suggesting alternatives; and in describing the neglect of foot health. The authors everywhere propose useful ways ahead. Their investigation for the best use of the chiropody manpower available is particularly interesting.

The DLF will do its utmost to secure consideration for the report, and to get it as widely read as possible. Much needs to be done in the way of further research to validate further the results of the enquiries. Nevertheless we have here a spring-board for action.

Problems Afoot:
Need and Efficiency in Footcare

Judith Kemp MSc SRCh MChS

J. T. Winkler MSc

Illustrations by Brenda Naylor

DISABLED LIVING FOUNDATION
London

First published in 1983

© Disabled Living Foundation
346 Kensington High Street
London W14 8NS

ISBN 0-901908-44-4

British Library Cataloguing in Publication Data
Kemp, Judith
    Problems afoot: need and efficiency in footcare.
    1. Foot—Care and hygiene
    I. Title   II. Winkler, J. T.
    617'.585   RD563

CONTENTS

Part V: Reforming Footcare: Policy and Practice 161

The DLF Trustees congratulate the authors warmly and will do all in their power to see that their original and constructive work gets the follow up it deserves.

W. M. Hamilton

LIST OF TABLES

List of Figures

Part I

Introduction: Problems, Concepts, Institutions

1 The problem: imbalanced need and provision

One of the major difficulties facing people who suffer from foot problems is to find someone who can help them. Theoretically, of course, everyone with foot trouble ought to be able to get help from the National Health Service (NHS). In practice, the situation is quite different. This book examines the problems involved in providing adequate footcare, and suggests ways of overcoming them.

The term 'footcare' covers all possible treatments given to the feet, from simple nail cutting to major surgical interventions. Care may be given by a correspondingly wide range of people, including the sufferers themselves, relatives, pedicurists, chiropodists, doctors, nurses, physiotherapists and surgeons, among others.

Despite this apparent profusion, so many people have problems with their feet that there are too few skilled people to give them the treatment they need. There are waiting lists alike for orthopaedic surgery and basic foot hygiene. Chiropodists, the specialists in foot problems, are in particularly short supply. As a result, the NHS has had to ration the chiropody services, restricting access to four 'priority groups' – elderly people, handicapped people, school children and expectant mothers. In practice, the service is unable to cope even with the demands made upon it by elderly people alone.

State of crisis

A state of crisis will be reached in the next decade because the number of elderly people (who have the most foot problems) is rising rapidly, the proportion of the total population aged over 65 is becoming larger and so is the number of people living beyond the age of 75. Yet elderly people are the group least able to look after their own feet, or to purchase treatment.

In the present economic climate, there is little likelihood of extra resources to expand services or to provide extra training places,

3

despite the recognition by successive governments that there is a real need for more chiropodists within the NHS. The problem then is of a growing number of potential patients, but restricted resources of both finance and skills. Conventionally, this might be described as an excess of demand over supply. But because of NHS rationing, many people with foot problems never get the chance to articulate demands; their needs remain unexpressed and unmet. Therefore, it is more accurate to describe the basic problem in footcare as a vast imbalance between the need for care and the provision of services.

Existing information about need

While professionals in footcare know that they are overwhelmed with calls for their services, surprisingly little factual information exists about the need for footcare. Foot health is essential for the mobility necessary to lead a full, normal life. Yet the only major survey into foot problems is *Trouble with feet* by May Clarke, a sociologist using chiropodists as research assistants to conduct foot examinations.

This is the principal source quoted and used by chiropodists for service planning. It gives valuable information about the number of people with foot trouble, but does not attempt to identify requirements for the various types of footcare. Moreover, chiropody has changed dramatically since the fieldwork was done in 1966.

The survey covered all age groups in 12 areas of the UK. Clarke estimated that 70 to 90% of people aged 65 and over had some trouble with their feet. Of these, at least half would benefit from chiropody treatment. This can be regarded as a rough estimate of need: 50% of those over 65.

In contrast, Peter Townsend and Dorothy Wedderburn in *The aged in the Welfare State* (1965) – a survey of all services provided by the State for elderly people – estimate that 30% of them needed chiropody. The people concerned did not have their feet examined, but were asked to describe their foot problems.

The difficulties of handicapped people were illustrated by M. D. Warren in *The Canterbury survey of handicapped people* (1974). Every household in Canterbury was visited to locate all handicapped people and determine their needs for, and receipt of, services such as meals on wheels, district nursing, chiropody, attendances at day centres, clubs, etc. Only 14% (107) were receiving chiropody treatment. Of these, 97 were elderly, most being over 75. A slightly larger number of people, whilst not in receipt of treatment, felt they required it. Thus, again, about 30% of handicapped people, by their own estimation, needed chiropody.

Part of the explanation for Clarke's higher assessment of need is that she used professional chiropodial examinations to establish need, while the other two studies relied on the subjects' own judgement.

These indicators of need for chiropody services are summarised in Table 1.

Table 1: Existing indicators of need for chiropody

	Elderly people	Handicapped people
In active receipt of service	7 – 18%	14%
Others who felt they needed the service	11%	14%
Total	18 – 29%	28%
Clinically assessed to be in need	50%	—

The discrepancy between the two figures for elderly people indicates that not all foot trouble is recognised by the people who suffer from it or they do not see it as treatable by a chiropodist.

These surveys did not attempt to differentiate between simple and more complex footcare needs. They do, however, show that there is unmet need for chiropody. The next section explores the likelihood of meeting that need.

The supply of chiropodists

Scant as our information may be on the need for footcare, there is even less on the provision of skills. The only detailed study of chiropodists is *A survey of manpower resources in the NHS chiropody service,* prepared by the Association of Chief Chiropody Officers (ACCO, 1980). Only chiropodists holding the officially-recognised qualification and listed in the State Register are eligible for employment in the NHS. The Register for 1979/80 listed 5,081 chiropodists. The ACCO survey showed that the NHS employed an equivalent of 2,570 full-time chiropodists – only a little over half those eligible. The rest work in private practice, industry or commerce.

As a basis for estimating the staff required to treat elderly people, the Society of Chiropodists and other professional bodies formulated a norm of one chiropodist per 1,000 elderly population. (Appendix II).

The ACCO survey demonstrated that the NHS region with the best ratio had only 0.43 chiropodists per 1,000 elderly population, a shortfall of 57%. The region with the worst ratio had only 0.10% chiropodists per 1,000 – a shortfall of 90%. Thus, patients have different chances of obtaining service, depending on where they live. But all NHS regions are short of chiropodists, even to serve this one group.

92.7% of the time of chiropodists employed in the NHS is spent in clinical work, 2.1% in making orthoses (permanent corrective/ palliative devices, e.g. insoles, latex dips), 4.2% in management, and 1% in all other activities, so it cannot be said that management deprives the NHS of much clinical time. Of the clinical and orthotic hours, 85.9% is spent on elderly people, 4.1% on handicapped people, 2.8% on children, 0.2% on expectant mothers and 6.9% on 'others' – probably mostly hospital patients. Two points are clear from these statistics. Elderly people are receiving most of the NHS chiropody service. But even if they were to receive all of it, there would still not be enough to meet the need. ACCO calculated that the NHS has less than half the chiropodists it needs to cope with elderly people alone. How many it would need to provide a comprehensive national service is beyond calculation because so little is known about the footcare needs of the general population.

The growth in numbers of state registered chiropodists is slow – 4,400 on the first Register in 1964, and only 5,319 in mid 1982. While the Schools of Chiropody have expanded wherever possible, their combined output of students is still only approximately 275 a year. However, 7% of the NHS chiropodists are over 60 and 28.5% over 50 years old. By 1994 the NHS will have lost 35.5% of its current (full-time equivalent) staff. Thus, there will be little increase in the total number of state registered chiropodists for the foreseeable future. While training facilities should be expanded wherever possible, this, by itself, will not overcome the problem of unmet need.

A response to the problem

To summarise, there is imbalance between need and provision in footcare, but information is lacking about both sides of the non-equation. Faced with this situation, the authors have tried to fill a few of those gaps, by investigating need among specific sections of the population and the quality of services provided to meet it.

The authors are a chiropodist practising in the National Health Service and a sociologist working in a university department of social policy. The study was designed as applied social research not merely to increase our intellectual understanding of footcare problems but also to find ways of overcoming them. This book sets out the facts discovered, draws out the implications, and goes on to make specific recommendations for changes in policy and practice, at both national and local levels, by everyone involved. There are sections for social workers and education authorities, the shoe trade, health administrators and health educators, nurses and doctors, voluntary foot carers as well as professionals. Therefore, the book is in no sense technical. Only so much of the physiology of the foot as is necessary for lay readers is described and only so much of the research methodology as is necessary for non-specialists to appreciate the significance of the results, including their limitations. Naturally, there is also a great deal to report to those professionally engaged in footcare, especially chiropodists. But the relevance of the research extends well beyond the experts.

Because the world of footcare is complex, ten separate studies were conducted within the overall project, five on need and five on provision. But although many people generously supported this project, limited resources of money, time and labour forced numerous restrictions and compromises on the work. Since the authors are robust in expressing their policy recommendations, they must be equally candid in explaining their limitations. Three were particularly important.

First, geographical coverage had to be restricted to one health district in inner London, an area that ranks high on all the traditional indicators of social deprivation, but which has both a chiropody service and a teaching hospital of high repute.

Second, groups to study had to be selected. For pragmatic reasons it was decided to focus on the needs of the four existing priority groups (elderly people, handicapped people, school children and expectant mothers), plus people on the waiting list for chiropody. A study of footcare need among the working population is necessary, but was well beyond the resources available. Among service providers, three types of doctors important in footcare were selected – surgeons, general practitioners, and casualty doctors/

departments. Because chiropodists are at the heart of footcare, two investigations of them were carried out.

Third, compromises were made in the scale and methods of the research. The techniques used were varied according to the groups studied – interviews, physical examinations, observation, documentary analysis and postal questionnaires. The specific methods used are described in the separate sections of the report along with the compromises that had to be made on the scale of the research. Sometimes it was possible to do a complete census of a group, but in other cases only small samples could be taken. The number of subjects covered could have been restricted, but the authors felt it was important to gather some information on both sides of the need/provision imbalance. Despite all its admitted limitations, this research will add substantially to the stock of knowledge about footcare: that is not a boast, it is a sad comment on the scarcity of existing information.

The book contains five sections covering (1) the important concepts and issues in footcare need and provision; (2) vulnerable patient groups – their particular problems – the research method used to study them, the findings and relevant policy recommendations; (3) the principal providers of services – under the same four headings; (4) the role of footwear in foot problems, and the changing role of chiropody as seen by chiropodists themselves; and (5) co-ordinated recommendations for reforms in policy and practice for each of the principal groups in the footcare world.

2 Need: potential, felt, activated

To outsiders, one of the most surprising characteristics of foot troubles is that the people who need care often do not realise it. This emerged clearly in the few available studies, described earlier. Even when people recognise that something is wrong with their feet, they may not actively seek treatment.

There are good physiological reasons behind this apparently curious behaviour. The shape of the feet may become deformed gradually over a period of years, so that people do not notice the changes and think that their feet were always 'naturally' this way. Similarly, it may take a long time to build up the lesions that eventually become painful and immobilising.

Even if people do not notice or act upon their foot problems at once, they will feel the pain sometime in the future and seek treatment. From the limited evidence available it seems likely that the current demand for treatment is only a small part of true need. Any serious attempt to assess the need for footcare, therefore, must take account of the full potential demand.

The authors attempted to do this by dividing the concept of need into three defined and measurable sub-categories: activated need, felt need and potential need.

Activated need: is a requirement for footcare which is consciously recognised by the sufferer or by a third party, and some action is taken to obtain relief.

Felt need: is a requirement for footcare which is consciously recognised by the sufferer or by a third party but no action is taken to obtain relief.

Potential need: is a requirement for footcare which is unrecognised by the individual or any third party. It would be recognised by a footcare professional in a clinical examination if one were carried out. It will remain potential until this happens or until the condition progresses and becomes felt need.

Table 2: The pyramid of need

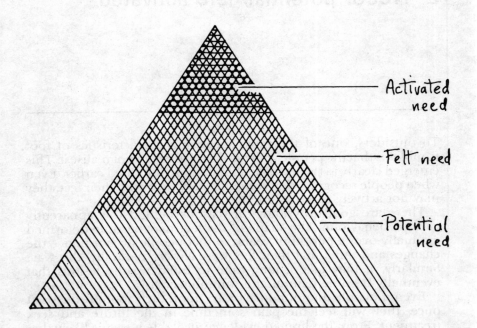

The bottom two tiers of the pyramid – felt and potential need – are only discovered by footcare professionals when either the condition becomes more acute and the sufferer is forced to seek help or the condition is detected by a third party. This may happen formally, as in child or geriatric screening programmes, or informally when, for some other reason, the feet are exposed to a relative or friend. Felt need and potential need are thus, by definition, unmet needs. Unmet need in elderly people is frequently discovered on their admission to hospital. Often, the person knows that something is wrong but has not sought help, perhaps through fear, ignorance or a feeling of shame for having let his or her feet get into such a neglected state.

Activated need, that which is recognised and acted upon, can be subdivided in several ways. Some people who request NHS chiropody do not receive it because they are put on a waiting list. Activated need thus includes some whose needs are unmet, as well as many whose needs are being provided for. The ways in which

Table 3: Multiple concepts of need

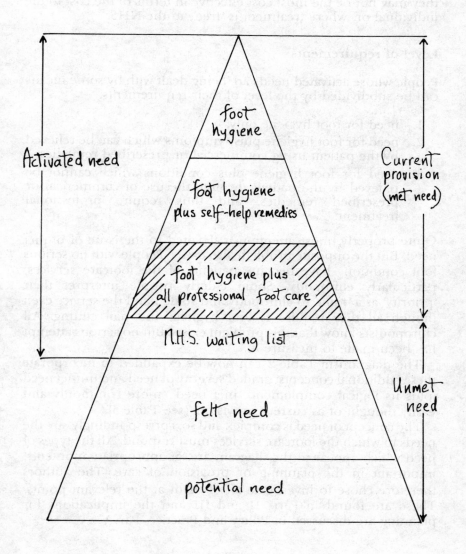

activated needs are dealt with may or may not be clinically effective; they may not be the most cost effective in terms of the cost to the individual or, where treatment is 'free', to the NHS.

Level of requirements

People whose activated needs are being dealt with by some means can be subdivided by the level of their requirements:

1. need for foot hygiene only;
2. need for foot hygiene plus symptoms which can be relieved by the patient using commercial or prescribed remedies;
3. need for foot hygiene plus conditions which cannot be relieved by the patient through the use of commercial or prescribed remedies, and thus require professional treatment.

Quite properly, most attention is devoted to the issue of unmet need. But the opposite problem also exists. People with no serious foot conditions have become patients of the footcare services, particularly chiropody. Some elderly people interpret their 'priority' as a 'right' to chiropody and so demand the service even though all they require is foot hygiene and nail cutting. All chiropodists know that this problem exists, but no serious attempt has been made to measure it.

The diagram in Table 2 can now be expanded to incorporate these additional concepts: graded severity of need and unmet need (plus its logical complement, 'met need', more commonly and easily thought of as current provision) (see Table 3).

The concept of need is complex and so, correspondingly, are the needs to which the footcare services must respond. All the types of need which appear in the diagram are, at appropriate moments, important in the planning or provision of care. The authors therefore chose to investigate all of them at the relevant points. These are found in Parts II and III and the implications for planning are discussed in Policy and Practice, Part V.

3 Provision: who delivers footcare?

The most basic form of footcare is self help. Basic hygiene and nail cutting may be all that is required to maintain the feet in good health. If not, many people purchase chiropody requisites, such as sponge insoles for comfort, insoles for insulation, arch supports, toe dividers or protectors, or other mechanical devices designed to relieve pressure, straighten toes, relieve strain, etc. Chemicals may also be purchased in the form of corn cures, either as plasters or liquids, medicated foot powders, creams or deodorants or anti-fungal preparations. A third group of commonly purchased items are the abrasives and cutters for hard skin (callous) removal. These range from pumice stone to the newer abrasive synthetic materials, which come in a variety of textures, through to corn knives and razor blades.

These commercial products may be more or less effective in dealing with the actual foot problem. In many cases, especially corns and callouses, the underlying cause of the lesion goes unrecognised and the lesions simply recur, so that only the symptom has been treated. In other conditions, such as fungal infections, diagnosed by a professional person, self help is the best method of cure, as the condition requires a once or twice daily application of an appropriate medication. However, for many people, self help, even with commercial remedies to assist, becomes inadequate and they seek assistance from another person, often a relative or close friend.

This may be satisfactory if the need is for simple foot hygiene (washing and nail cutting) only. If no-one is willing to help or the foot condition is beyond the skill of a friend or relative, help must be sought from professional people either in the NHS or the private sector.

The public sector

A wide range of professional personnel within the NHS may offer footcare treatment in one form or another: nurses, doctors – both family and hospital – surgeons, physiotherapists and chiropodists are the major groups. Whilst each is a separate, recognised profession with its own area of expertise, their scope of practice overlaps in important ways.

Nurses

Nurses may, for this purpose, be divided into three groups: district nurses, hospital nurses and school nurses. District nurses cut toenails for patients and refer only those with more complex foot problems. Hospital nurses also cut toenails as part of basic care. Admission to hospital may provide the first opportunity for an elderly person's foot problems to be discovered and, if necessary, referred. School nurses have the opportunity to screen children's feet at a crucial stage.

Family doctors

For most of the population, however, their first resort is not the hospital but their family doctor (general practitioner – GP). Many foot problems are treated by GPs but it is unrealistic to expect them to be experts in everything. Moreover, many foot conditions are unimportant when compared with the potentially-life threatening conditions presented, so GPs may not refer or even recognise as many foot conditions as they might.

Hospitals

When GPs do refer problems, it is usually to hospital. However, a hospital consists of many departments including physicians who specialise in diabetes, skin or arthritic conditions, surgeons who specialise in orthopaedic or vascular surgery, physiotherapists and chiropodists. Patients may also be referred – or refer themselves – to the Accident and Emergency (Casualty) department where they may be treated or referred to a specialist.

Physiotherapists

Physiotherapists, who are principally concerned with the deeper structures, especially muscles, ligaments and bones, aim to restore or improve the function of these structures. In regard to the feet and legs they treat such injuries as sprains and strains, and work with patients who have limited use of a limb through strokes, accidents, or illness. Their role is thus one of rehabilitation. They may treat scars which are troublesome but they do not treat other common skin lesions such as corns and callouses.

Chiropodists

Chiropodists specialise in the treatment of the leg and foot. Their knowledge extends beyond the foot itself as many of its problems are related to particular systemic diseases or disorders. Chiropodists diagnose foot problems and give appropriate treatments, not the least important part of which is in advising patients how they can help themselves and the chiropodist. This frequently involves footwear advice, which may prevent the onset of a condition or help in a cure. The conditions diagnosed and treated can range from damaged toe nails, corns and callouses (all quite common), to disorders of cartilage in a child's foot, sprains, stress fractures and mechanical instability. Chiropodists can deal with minor infections, those which do not require antibiotics and most soft tissue injuries not requiring sutures. They also, where they hold the necessary certificate, use injectable local analgesics, which allows them to undertake avulsions (removal) of toe nails.

They can also diagnose other conditions which require treatment by doctors or surgeons. The chiropodist, not infrequently, is the first to recognise diseases which affect the whole body, but have manifestations in the feet, since the chiropodist may be the only person with any medical training with whom the patient has regular contact. Finally, there are many foot conditions which the chiropodist would treat in conjuction with the patient's doctor. Because chiropodists are so central to footcare, their scope of practice overlaps the skills of all the other professionals involved.

Private sector providers of footcare

Footcare treatments can be obtained outside the NHS: from private chiropodists, pedicurists, beauty therapists and reflexologists as well as private doctors.

Private chiropodists have a similar scope of practice to those in the NHS but as the training of chiropodists as a whole varies widely, detailed discussion will be found in Chapter 5.

Beauty therapists and pedicurists offer a range of feet 'treatments' which include nail cutting and varnishing, foot massage and hard skin removal. Their knowledge of feet will vary according to their training (if any). However, they provide a service which is satisfactory to some consumers.

Reflexologists claim to be able to diagnose and, in some cases, cure bodily diseases by massaging the foot at a particular point which is supposed to represent the diseased organ. It is an ancient art, supposedly working in the same way as acupuncture.

Private doctors offer treatment to feet as do private physio-therapists, especially for sports injuries, on an unknown, but growing scale.

It can be seen, then, that a number of occupational groups with a range of skills, participate in the provision of footcare. The next Chapter examines in detail the matching of problems to skills in what is called the 'Footcare Spectrum'.

4 The footcare spectrum: problems and skills in parallel

When people with foot problems seek help three things may happen:

(i) they may receive the help they need;

(ii) they may be referred on, because their conditions require a higher level of skill than that possessed by the person approached;

(iii) they may be turned away, because what is required is too simple to merit the skills of a specialist.

A choice between these three options faces all providers of treatment – doctors, chiropodists, pedicurists, relatives. An example might make this clear.

An elderly man has a badly deformed and thickened nail which is making it difficult to wear shoes. He is in good health, but cannot bend to reach his foot and asks his niece to cut the nail. She attempts the task, but cannot manage. The condition is beyond her skill (ii above). The man then turns to his general practitioner for help. The GP may have had experience in cutting these difficult nails and, if he has suitable nail clippers, may do the job himself (i above). If not, he may refer the patient to someone who can (ii above). Or, he might consider that nail cutting is not a proper use of his time and training. He might therefore decline treatment and refer the man on (iii above).

Whomever the man was referred to, the treatment technique (and, it is hoped, also the outcome) would be similar, but the GP's choice of referral would be more or less costly to the NHS depending on whether he selected a hospital department or a chiropodist. If the patient was sent to a hospital, he might find, yet again, that the doctor in the Accident and Emergency Department thought nail cutting a waste of his time and skill, especially if there was a chiropodist available to whom he could refer the man further.

From this it becomes apparent that, for everyone involved in the footcare world, there may be three groups of patients; those within their scope of practice, those beyond it and those who could be adequately treated by someone less highly trained. This can be illustrated using registered chiropodists as the professional group.

1. Sub-chiropodial needs: conditions which may be adequately treated by persons with less training and skill than a registered chiropodist, e.g. a need for foot hygiene and normal nail cutting.

2. Chiropodial needs: conditions which cannot be adequately treated by people with less training than a registered chiropodist, e.g. a need for cure and further prevention of ulcers on the sole of foot.

3. Supra-chiropodial needs: conditions which cannot be treated even by registered chiropodists as they require skills beyond their scope of practice, e.g. grafting of bones in the foot after injury.

The chiropodial and sub-chiropodial needs could, of course, also be treated by others more highly trained than chiropodists, for example doctors. But this would be doubly wasteful. First, the cost to the NHS of identical treatment would be higher, simply because the time of doctors is more expensive than the time of chiropodists. Second, the doctors could have been treating other cases which did require their training and expertise.

Ideally, the cost-effectiveness of the NHS would be improved if every patient was dealt with by the professional who is competent, but not overqualified, to treat the condition in question.

However, that presumes that patients and professionals could be readily classified. Lots of things can go wrong with feet. They can also be affected by disorders of nerves, muscles and circulation, body chemistry (e.g. diabetes) and many diseases. Any problem with the hips or spine which affects the way in which a person walks will affect the feet. The many possible combinations of conditions make an unambiguous classification of foot patients difficult.

Similarly, as mentioned earlier, the scope of practice of many professions overlaps with that of others. And, within each profession, there will be differences of skill. Thus, in practice, specific problems do not fall tidily within, beyond or beneath each group's skill.

The efficient linking of patients to professionals is not easy. But the waste through using expensive personnel to treat simple foot conditions can be large. In the pedestrian matters of the NHS, it is worth trying to fit means to ends.

Footcare may be thought of as the collection of all the skills, techniques and treatments which are employed to maintain or

Table 4: The footcare spectrum

Major orthopaedic surgery —
 e.g. to fix ankle in one position.
Operations for bunions.
Operations to straighten lesser toes.
Operations to excise toenails and
 growth area.
Other procedures to remove nails and
 sterilise growth area:
Treatments to correct foot function —
 e.g. excessive laxity or rigidity at joints.
Treatment for correction of deformities —
 e.g curly toes in children.
Treatments for soft tissues —
 e.g. ulcers, strains.
Treatments for infections —
 e.g. fungal infections, warts.
Treatments for palliation of bony deformities —
 e.g. bunions, hammer toes.
Treatments for skin lesions —
 e.g. corns, callouses.
Treatments for nails —
 e.g. thinning of thickened nails.
Foot hygiene for those who cannot manage —
 e.g. the blind, those who cannot grip.
Nail cutting of normal nails.

supra chiropody

chiropody

sub chiropody

restore foot health, including normal feet, as well as those affected
by accident or deformity. A normal foot is one which performs all
the functions which may be expected of it in walking, running,
climbing, etc., without pain.

The simplest form of footcare is the washing and drying of the
feet in order to maintain the skin in a healthy condition, plus the
cutting of the nails. Very complex, in contrast, are the major
operations carried out by orthopaedic surgeons to correct or repair
damage to the bone structure of the feet. In between these two
extremes are a vast number of conditions requiring differing types
of care, which may be set out along a spectrum of increasing
severity. Parallel, we may align the continuum of skills appropriate
to dealing with them. Together they make the footcare spectrum.
The concept is illustrated in Table 4.

In the centre of the spectrum is a band which may be considered
'chiropody'. But the position and width of that band are the subject
of controversy. The idea that some skills may be supra-chiropodial
and others sub-chiropodial is clear in theory, but the boundaries
have never been very sharp and recently they have been changing.
The complexity of present-day chiropody requires further
explanation.

5 Chiropody: ambiguity and change

The purpose of this chapter is to explain to non-specialist readers the nature of chiropody and the various types of chiropodists. It is not, however, just a technical prologue. Ambiguity of definition is one of the central problems in footcare.

The term 'chiropody' has always covered a wide range of treatments. That range has increased over the past decade through improvements in training. As a result, there are few people outside the profession who know the full scope of competence possessed by a fully trained chiropodist today. Most members of the general public and indeed most other health professionals underestimate the capacity of chiropody, feeling that it is mainly concerned with cutting corns and nails.

The uncertainty and underestimation create practical difficulties. The relationship of chiropody to the other footcare services remains ill-defined, and hence, the allocation of patients between them haphazard.

In practice, most other professionals act conservatively, sending chiropodists only a narrow range of patients with relatively minor problems. The public, also, tend to seek little more than basic foot hygiene. As a result the chiropody service becomes overloaded with routine, low-skill work. Patients with more serious foot problems cannot get access to the service, chiropodists' more advanced skills go unused, and morale sinks.

Thus, defining chiropody is a practical policy problem. This book cannot give a firm, short answer to that question, but seeks to clarify the present ambiguity and point out its implications. What is at issue is the organisation of footcare.

What is chiropody?

Attempts at definitions have usually been descriptions of the work commonly then being undertaken. Current official and popular definitions are both wide of the mark. The Chiropodists Board of

21

the Council for the Professions Supplementary to Medicine has written that 'Chiropody comprises the maintenance of the feet in healthy condition, and the treatment of their disabilities by recognised chiropodial methods in which the practitioner has been trained'. This fits state registered chiropodists, who have undergone a standard training and passed the appropriate examinations. But it does not cover the work done by several thousand others, since, under the present law, anyone can set up in practice and call himself a chiropodist without any training at all. By contrast, that traditional source of popular definitions, the *Concise Oxford Dictionary*, accurately reflects the way most people underestimate the scope of present-day chiropody: 'Chiropody: treatment given to feet, esp. for corns, bunions, etc'.

The problem can be approached by a more sophisticated route, using the Footcare Spectrum (Table 4). Clearly, chiropody lies somewhere in the middle of the range of skills appropriate for dealing with foot problems. But where exactly are the upper and lower boundaries? That is, what treatments can and should chiropodists provide?

An important decision has to be made in defining the lower boundary of chiropody. Most people keep their feet clean and nails trimmed, but others, particularly elderly people, very much want (or need) this done for them. The issue is: should chiropodists be undertaking this foot hygiene? After their expensive three-year training, it is a costly way to give basic footcare. And in the present state of excess demand, every patient they accept for foot hygiene means denying another patient with more serious foot problems.

If chiropodists decline to do this type of work, some other provision must be made for those who cannot do it for themselves. Foot hygiene for healthy adults could be carried out by many others. But foot hygiene for people with some relatively common conditions, e.g. impaired circulation, should still be done by a trained professional. Determining whether the adult is 'healthy' however, is often a difficult decision, particularly in the case of elderly patients. This adds another complication to the issue of whether foot hygiene is part of 'chiropody' or 'sub-chiropody'.

The boundary between 'chiropody' and 'supra chiropody' is also debatable. The training of state registered chiropodists now includes the use of injectable local analgesics which means that much more advanced work can be undertaken.

Whilst much of this advanced work is merely an extension of treatments traditionally associated with chiropody, the ability to suppress pain does, theoretically, make it possible for chiropodists to move into new areas of work. This possibility is viewed with suspicion by some doctors, whilst others positively approve.

There is also debate among chiropodists themselves. Those who have qualified recently have a different outlook from those trained years ago. The competence of chiropodists is increasing. Should the boundaries of chiropody move upwards correspondingly?

Who are chiropodists?

Chiropodists are the specialists of the problems of the foot but their degree of skill varies widely. In the United Kingdom, anyone can set up in practice as a 'chiropodist', advertise and charge unrestricted fees for treatment given. There is no mandatory examination of skill and therefore no minimum level of training. There is no inspection of work and claims of malpractice have to be pursued through civil law. In some areas a licence may be required under local bye-laws, but this only licences the premises, not the practitioner. At the other extreme, an officially recognised course of training must be undertaken and passed if a chiropodist wishes to work for the National Health Service. Thus, one important way of subdividing chiropodists is between those who have completed the officially recognised training and those who have not.

State registered chiropodists

The recognised training of chiropodists is carried out at 11 Schools of Chiropody in the United Kingdom. This part of the profession is regulated by the Council for Professions Supplementary to Medicine (CPSM) along with other professions such as occupational therapy, physiotherapy and radiography. The syllabus of training and the examinations are set by the Society of Chiropodists on behalf of the Chiropodists Board. The course is for three years of full-time study; professional examinations are taken at the end of each year, passes in all subjects being required.

The chiropodist is thereby equipped to diagnose and treat virtually all foot conditions which do not require systemic drugs, stitching of tendons or skin wounds or internal fixation (such as plating fractures). Diagnosis is frequently possible even where treatment is beyond the scope of practice. Chiropodists who have passed the examination are now able to obtain and inject local analgesics (anaesthetics) in order to use techniques requiring the suppression of pain, such as some more radical treatments for plantar warts *(verrucae)* and ingrowing toenails. Both conditions can also be treated without local analgesia but with different techniques.

Successful completion of the course and examinations makes the person eligible for entry as a state registered chiropodist (SRCh) on the State Register published annually by the Chiropodists Board. Registration is required for employment in the NHS, but not in private practice. A fee is paid annually to retain one's name on the Register; no re-examination of competence is required. On the inception of the Register, provision was made to include chiropodists who, whilst not having a recognised qualification, had experience in the field and met certain other criteria laid down in the Professions Supplementary to Medicine Act 1960. The first Register, published in 1964, listed 4,400 chiropodists. By mid-1982, there were 5,319, an expansion of less than 1% a year. It is an offence under the PSM Act 1960 to use the description 'state registered chiropodist', 'registered chiropodist' or 'state chiropodist' if not on the current Register, but there is no restriction on using the word 'chiropodist' itself.

Non state registered chiropodists

This group may be divided into two sub-sections: (1) those who are eligible for, but who are not currently on, the State Register; and (2) those who are not eligible for entry on the State Register.

No systematic information is available on either of these groups. Although several associations represent non-registered chiropodists, their coverage is not complete, their memberships overlap, and they publish no lists. No research has been done on their skills, location, patients or fees. There is not even a reliable estimate of numbers. The first group is probably quite small, since it is usually advantageous to maintain state registration. For the others, estimates range from 2,500 to 10,000. A recent postal advertising campaign by a commercial firm located approximately 11,000 chiropodists, implying just under 6,000 non-registered. But there is no way of knowing the thoroughness of the coverage.

The training of non-registered chiropodists varies greatly. A few have completed the recognised three-year course. Others have undertaken substantial training programmes of varying length. Still others have learned through correspondence courses, which sometimes include a practical component. Some have effectively done an informal apprenticeship through working with another non-registered chiropodist. Some other health professionals, especially nurses, have become involved in footcare during the course of their other work and decided to work in chiropody, without having any specialist training.

It is only partially possible for an intending patient or others to learn about the training of chiropodists. Only state registered chiropodists may work in the NHS. State registered chiropodists working in the private sector will be listed in the annual register, which is available for inspection at public reference libraries. There is no published information on the individual training of non-registered chiropodists.

The possible combinations of qualification and employment in chiropody are summarised in the following table.

Table 5: Qualifications and employment in chiropody

	National Health Service	Private Practice
Registered	Only registered may work for the NHS. May work full-time, but many work only part-time.	Full-time private practitioner does not need registration but may maintain it in order to do part-time work in or for the NHS.
Non Registered	Excluded by regulations under the NHS Act.	Large, but unknown numbers, variable levels of training.

Footcare assistants (FCAs)

In a decision that was to have extended repercussions for all types of chiropodists, the Department of Health and Social Security introduced a new grade of foot health worker in 1977, the footcare assistant (FCA). The Department explained the rationale and content of the role in Circular (HC(77)9) which contains the following paragraphs.

'5.   Part of a trained chiropodist's time is spent on work which does not require his skills and expertise but which cannot be undertaken by the patients themselves. For the elderly, arthritic and other handicapped persons, the blind and the partially sighted, this type of work can be done by supportive staff (footcare assistants). Employment of such staff would reduce the cost to the NHS of present levels of treatment and facilitate extension of chiropody services as envisaged in "Priorities for Health and Personal Social Services" and the Department's planning guidelines.

'6. The tasks they might carry out include simple footcare and hygiene, such as the cutting of toenails. Their training should be undertaken under the direction of the Area Chiropodist and would normally be on the basis of in-service instruction given by a fulltime NHS chiropodist. They should receive instruction not only in the tasks they are to perform but also in recognising conditions that require the attention of a state registered chiropodist. The extent or degree of supervision of footcare assistants would depend on local circumstances and should be left to the discretion of the supervising chiropodist. In two chair clinics, for example, they might most usefully be employed in assisting a chiropodist by preparing patients and carrying out simple and preparatory work. Before being treated by supportive staff all persons should be seen first by a qualified chiropodist who would decide whether the patient's condition could be attended to by such staff and would specify any care required. The chiropodist should himself see such patients at intervals'.

Footcare assistants were thus seen as low cost labour for low skill tasks. The developing crisis in footcare made this seem a reasonable innovation from the Department's point of view. The demand for chiropody, particularly from elderly people was increasing rapidly and was likely to expand still further as the numbers of elderly people themselves rose throughout the remainder of this century. In contrast, the number of state registered chiropodists was growing only very slowly. Even if the training schools were expanded rapidly, demand for footcare would never be met by this means alone. So what the Department decided was effectively to divide the work chiropodists currently do into two parts: foot hygiene and genuine chiropody. It then created a new grade of worker, with very brief training and a lower salary, to take over the hygiene part of the job.

Whatever the good intentions of the DHSS, the innovation was resisted by the profession. The notion of an assistant to do the repetitive, less interesting work and to help generally was naturally welcome, but under the regulations promulgated by the DHSS there was no definition of the scope of practice for footcare assistants, nor was there a firm requirement that they should work under direct supervision of a fully-qualified chiropodist. In consequence, there was nothing to stop FCAs gaining as much experience as they could within the NHS and then setting up in private practice. This possibility generated opposition in many parts of the profession. Registered chiropodists did not like the idea of being asked to train FCAs who might then call themselves 'chiropodists'. Others in the private sector did not like the idea of creating a substantial new group of potential competitors.

As a result, one of the professional associations, the Society of Chiropodists, issued a letter in July 1977 to all its members and employing authorities in the United Kingdom on the subject (*The Chiropodist*, Vol. 32, No. 9, Sept. 1977). It stated:

'In the view of the Society footcare assistants should only be used to cut the normal nails of patients who are unable to do it for themselves because of blindness or some other disability. There should be no need for training since all that needs to be done is:
1 clean the foot with a sachet of skin preparation
2 cut and file the nails, and
3 clean again with a sachet of skin preparation.'

The letter added that FCAs should only be employed where there are a minimum of two chairs in the clinic, and that a registered chiropodist be readily available during the procedure. In the April 1978 volume of the Society's journal, *The Chiropodist*, (Vol. 33, No. 4), further comment was made on the position of NHS staff who were members of the Society if asked to work with FCAs beyond the Society guidelines. This included the following: 'Should there be any abnormality, or should the patient be suffering from any medical or surgical condition likely to affect the foot, we (the Society) would expect the patient to be treated by a state registered chiropodist only'.

The Society's response was thus a complex one. It was not opposing footcare assistants outright. Indeed, it recognised that they are here to stay by recommending a ratio of 1 FCA to 6 chiropodists for NHS health authorities. Rather, by its guidelines the Society was trying to define and restrict the work the new assistants would be allowed to do. However, by interpreting these guidelines strictly, it is possible to exclude many elderly people from treatment. And since the elderly represent most of the NHS patients, this would severely limit the number of FCAs who could be used. In practice, this is what has happened. In January 1979, when the ACCO Manpower Survey was conducted, there were no FCAs in Wales, Scotland or Northern Ireland and only 52.6 were recorded in England. The attempt by the DHSS to create a new type of sub-chiropodial role has been effectively blocked.

Nonetheless, many registered chiropodists in the public sector accept that there is a need for foot hygiene as provided by FCAs and a good economic case for their introduction. Indeed they would be keen to release some of their caseload, in order to have the time for treating more complex foot conditions, if the objections could be overcome. This feeling led to a counter-proposal to the DHSS – closure of the profession.

Professional closure

Closure of the profession means restricting the right to practise as a chiropodist to people with specified qualifications. As one might expect in an occupation with as varied training arrangements as chiropody, the issue of closure has been the subject of debate for many years. A Statutory Instrument (1964 No. 940) effectively closed the practice within the public sector, while leaving the private sector unrestricted.

The introduction of footcare assistants intensified discussion about the subject. The most tangible result of this renewed interest was the issue of a Consultative Document by the DHSS in late 1981. This defined two possible forms of closure:

Functional closure – would restrict the right to practice to those who are state registered.

Indicative closure – would restrict the use of certain professional titles to those who are state registered.

It was made clear by the DHSS that functional closure was unlikely to be granted because it would limit the provision of chiropody to a small number of practitioners and thus restrict the availability to the public. Indicative closure on the other hand, 'would give the public the means of distinguishing between registered and unregistered practitioners, but unlike functional closure, it would not restrict the services available'.

Following further consultation with the professional associations, the DHSS decided that, because of a lack of consensus, no further legislation would be enacted for the time being. Thus, at the time of writing, the linked issues of footcare assistants and professional closure are in stalemate. Neither the Department nor the profession has got what it wants. But the issues will not go away. The chiropody service is already rationed, but still overloaded, while demand is rising rapidly and likely to grow still more. The crisis is approaching quickly. Some resolution will have to be negotiated. Some chiropody managers are going ahead without waiting for a settlement, introducing footcare assistants as they see fit. This theme is returned to repeatedly throughout the book.

Employment opportunities: private practice

One of the attractions of chiropody as a career, for some, is the prospect of being self-employed. Both state registered and non-registered chiropodists can treat patients without referral from a medical practitioner. Both may open a private practice where the patient pays a fee for each consultation. Registered chiropodists are subject to a strict code of ethics regarding advertising and announcements of commencement of practice, but this does not apply to the un-registered.

Many private practices are only part-time, the chiropodist having another regular source of income which may or may not be related to the practice of chiropody. Some private practitioners do not maintain any practice facilities at all, working only on a domiciliary basis. The chiropodist then only needs a visiting case which contains all his instruments, adhesive pads, strappings, antiseptics, etc. Working in this way is obviously much easier and less expensive than starting up an actual practice. It does require transport since the chiropodist has to go to the patient, not *vice versa*. However, it makes possible flexible working hours and combination with another job.

The registered chiropodist in private practice also has the chance of supplementary employment. Sessional work (i.e. for a three hour period) is available both within the NHS and in many industries. This is frequently an attractive proposition as industrial sessions present a varied mix of patients, all of working age. In NHS work, the majority of patients are elderly. Another alternative for the registered chiropodist is to become an NHS contractor. This is a system by which the Health Authority can send NHS patients to a local private practice, paying a fee for each treatment given. In this way the patients still receive free treatment as they would in an NHS clinic. For the non-registered, there are few alternatives for chiropodial employment outside their own private practice. Part-time work in the NHS is not open to them, though voluntary organisations and some commercial organisations do employ non-registered chiropodists.

Structure of NHS chiropody services

The structure of NHS chiropody services is quite complex. Most health authorities have a tripartite service, providing chiropody in the community, in hospitals, and on a domiciliary basis. Some rural authorities have mobile clinics in caravans which can be towed to outlying villages, giving the chiropodist excellent working facilities. Chiropody surgeries are now too sophisticated to be set up in a village hall and too expensive to be provided permanently where usage is small. A mobile clinic provides a practical alternative, and the towing vehicle can also be used to collect less ambulant patients. Caravans can also be used for visits to schools or old people's homes where facilities for chiropody are limited. The district may also use the contractor system, sending patients to a local private practice as described above. This is cost-effective in localities where the patient might otherwise require transport or a domiciliary visit. Contractors may also be used where recruitment is difficult because of the shortage of chiropodists.

The scarcity of state registered chiropodists has also led to one of the most important characteristics of the present day chiropody services, the priority group system. The DHSS recognises that there are not enough chiropodists to allow unrestricted access to NHS treatment. A circular (HRC74/33) issued during the reorganisation of the health service in 1974 states that 'in general treatment should continue to be restricted to the existing priority groups, viz. the elderly, the handicapped, expectant mothers and children still at school'. In theory, this system does not debar other patients, but in practice only a very small percentage of NHS chiropodists' time is spent on anyone other than patients from the priority groups. In effect, it is a rationing system.

But it is also a rationing system of an unusual type, with important consequences for chiropody and chiropodists. Attempts during the research to trace with the DHSS the origins and rationales for these groups proved fruitless. Probably the system was devised to concentrate treatment on those people whose needs were thought to be greatest. But what the DHSS did was to grant priority to whole categories of people rather than on the basis of need for chiropody. This created uncertainty whether access to treatment depended on one's membership of a social group or the condition of one's feet. Certainly many people now believe that elderly people have a 'right' to chiropody rather than simply first call on available services. This has led to a very skewed pattern of chiropody treatments. The diagram in Table 6 illustrates the amount of clinical time spent nationally on each of the priority groups and on all others.

Table 6: Distribution of chiropodists' clinical time

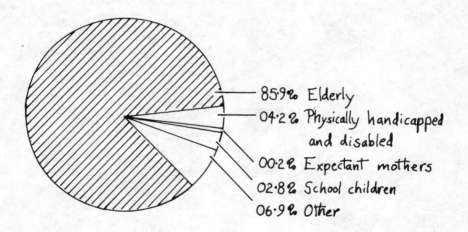

85·9% Elderly
04·2% Physically handicapped and disabled
00·2% Expectant mothers
02·8% School children
06·9% Other

Elderly people receive the overwhelming proportion of chiropody, far more than any other priority group. And all other patients receive not just lower priority for treatment, but very little treatment at all.

The predominance of elderly people has further consequences. Many of the conditions from which elderly patients suffer are due to underlying skeletal damage which cannot now be cured. All chiropodists can do is offer palliative treatments. This means that the range of skills in daily use by NHS chiropodists is rather narrow and towards the bottom of the footcare spectrum. And what is not part of the diagram, but equally important, the heavy load of routine treatment for elderly people means there is little time for preventive work.

In sum, the priority group system has a dominating influence on what chiropodists do. It is a crucial factor in the current problems in the footcare services.

6 An introduction to the foot: development and problems

Most patients who come to the footcare services are elderly. The young seldom complain about their feet. It is usually with advancing age that people become sensitive to the problems of their feet and begin to seek treatment. The reason lies in the natural development of the foot.

At birth, the 26 bones in the foot are basically represented by cartilage which is relatively soft and pliable. As the child grows, the areas of bone increase until, between the ages of 16 to 20, the bones of the foot are fully developed and the cartilage has disappeared except for the surfaces of the joints.

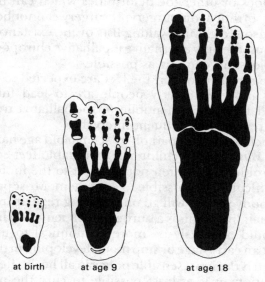

at birth   at age 9   at age 18

Fig. 1: Foot growth.

This process of conversion from cartilage to bone during growth is known as ossification. The resultant bone assumes the shape of the cartilage which it replaces. Cartilage is relatively soft and can be moulded quite painlessly by pressure. This is a useful phenomenon in the growing child as the skeleton can adapt to particular stresses while the cartilage is slowly turned to bone. It is when this process is completed that people stop growing. However, when young feet are put into hose or shoes which do not fit, this painless remodelling may cause a toe to curl or burrow under, or rise over its neighbour because there is no room for it to lie flat. Unless corrected, the toe will ossify in its new shape and position and may cause loss of function later in life. In childhood it is possible to use the malleability of cartilage to mould the toes back again.

Toes which are misshapen but still mobile may not cause pain, but with the onset of arthritis, common in feet, these toes may develop corns and callouses because the skin is subjected to intolerable pressure and friction. In addition, a reduction in function may be tolerable while the foot is sufficiently mobile to compensate, but when the foot becomes stiffer with age, this functional loss becomes noticeable. By then, correction by manipulation is not possible and the patient is left with hammer toes, curly toes or other toe deformities which can then only be corrected by orthopaedic surgery. If surgery cannot be performed for some reason (e.g. long waiting lists or the existence of medical complications) the only alternative is palliative chiropody, to give as much function and comfort as possible.

As people now live longer, the feet are expected to function for many years more. If elderly people are to lead full lives, it is important that they remain mobile. So the palliative treatments are commonly repeated at frequent intervals.

Thus, much of the foot pathology seen in old age has its origin in childhood. But because children's mouldable feet so rarely give pain, the problems are often not brought to the footcare services until it is difficult or impossible to cure them. Most patients of the NHS chiropody service will go on receiving regular treatments for the rest of their lives. This is a burden on patients and health service alike. It would obviously be more economical to intercept foot problems at an early stage or stop them developing in the first place.

Prevention is the most sensible policy in all health fields. But with many conditions it is at least possible to cure the problem and restore normality by medical intervention at a later stage. With foot pathology, this is often not the case, and prevention is the only sensible policy. An essential part of prevention is some method of detecting emergent foot problems in young people. The shortage of chiropodists makes it unlikely   that they could carry out an extensive screening programme on their own. However, since school nurses inspect feet as part of the annual School Health Service hygiene examination, a potential screening mechanism already exists. One study was designed, in part, to examine how well this service was working.

There are many problems which might be detected, with varied implications for the treatment services. When non-specialists envisage foot problems, it is usually corns, callouses and infections which come to mind. While these skin problems are important and often painful, skeletal and functional problems are the cardinal elements in foot pathology. These are dealt with first.

Knees, posture and gait

Knock knees, bow legs and abnormal gait can all be detected quite easily. Most knock knees and bow legs correct spontaneously and treatment is only given in severe cases which should have been diagnosed before the child started school. An abnormal gait can be a sign of hip trouble or underlying neurological problems, such as cerebral palsy or spina bifida. These too, should be detected before school age. All can, however, lead to foot problems or to difficulty with shoes, on which a chiropodist may be able to help.

Movements at joints

A range of movements at any joint may be considered normal. Limitation of the range or excessive laxity can cause problems requiring further advice or treatment. This may take the form of stretching to increase range, or exercise to strengthen the muscles. In some cases, further medical investigation may be required to eliminate systemic diagnoses. Chiropodists may prescribe and manufacture orthoses to limit the range of movement in some cases.

Whole foot deformities

The conditions of importance are club feet of any kind, very high arched or 'cavus' feet, and 'flat' feet of a particular sort. All these conditions would require supervision by an orthopaedic surgeon, even if surgery were not indicated immediately. But equally all can benefit from corrective or palliative insoles and shoe modifications advised by a chiropodist. Many children appear to have flat feet, especially in the early years. Most do not need treatment. The flat feet which require investigation are those which do not function normally – the rigid or painful ones. A quick test for rigid flat feet is to ask the child to stand on tip toe, with the back to the examiner. If the arch appears, then the foot is posturally (that is, naturally) flat. If it is painfree, it can be considered to be within the range of normality.

Forefoot deformities

Some of these are thought to be the result of molding whilst in the womb, e.g. *metatarsus varus*. In this condition, the forefoot is swung inwards in relation to the hindfoot, giving a more 'banana' shaped footprint than normal. It is a condition which usually corrects spontaneously, possibly helped by correctly fitting footwear.

Hallux valgus (bunion) is the most common problem associated with the great toe. It can be inherited or acquired through badly fitting footwear. It is difficult to pinpoint an exact cause in many cases but in Britain, where women's shoes are often more fashionable than healthy, women are far more likely to have bunions than men.

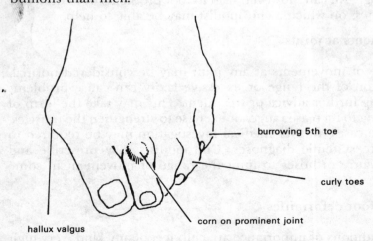

burrowing 5th toe

curly toes

corn on prominent joint

hallux valgus

Fig. 2: Forefoot deformities

Bunions are the opposite of spontaneously self correcting; once they start they tend to get worse. The musculature is arranged in such a way that, once the toe has altered its angle beyond a critical point, the muscles tend to pull the toe even further out of alignment. Whilst it is virtually impossible to correct *hallux valgus* without surgery, is obviously possible to reduce the extrinsic factors which accelerate the process. Badly fitting footwear, too narrow across the toes or not having a straight inner edge, can push the toe out of alignment and thus accelerate a process which might have happened anyway. On the other hand, footwear may trigger a process which would not have happened otherwise. Attention to footwear would obviously not prevent inherited *hallux valgus,* but it could be of value if it delayed the process allowing the feet to develop to the maximum first.

There are four toe deformities which may pass unnoticed in childhood, but which frequently lead to corns and callosities, and thus to much pain in later life.

1. Over-riding toes

There is a recognised congenital condition in which the little toe is retracted, that is, completely out of contact with the ground. This apparently causes little problem except in shoe fitting. Other toes, especially the second, may over-ride, either from birth or as a result from *hallux valgus.*

2. Curly toes

Many babies are born with toes that don't lie flat – but these generally straighten when the child begins to walk. The toe may be simply curled under, or it may curl sideways as well; the latter is probably most important in terms of foot function.

3. Hammer toes

These are toes in which the first joint in the toe itself becomes fixed, causing it to be more prominent than the other toes. It is commonly the second toe, especially where this is longer than the great toe.

4. Burrowing toes

These are toes which lie under the next toe. Burrowing 5th (little) toes are the most common, probably due to ill-fitting shoes and hose.

Some deformed toes are due to hereditary factors and some to intrinsic factors such as the position of muscle insertions, which means that attempts at correction by non-surgical methods will be doomed to failure. However, poor footwear may hasten the onset or speed of development of hereditary predispositions and some toe deformities may be due to moulding by inadequate footwear alone. These will be reversible before growth is completed. Prevention, by education in the correct way to buy and fit socks and shoes, could reduce the incidence of deformities caused by these factors.

Infections

There are two common infections of the feet. The *verruca* (wart) is found more often in children. *Verrucae* are virus infections of the skin, and may appear on any part of the foot. They vary in appearance and size, but those on areas of skin which take weight, or where shoes press on them, are often more painful. Chiropodists use a variety of treatments, ranging from adhesive plaster, through the use of acids in the form of pastes or paints, to freezing or electro-dessication, the latter under local anaesthetic. All treatments aim to kill the affected skin cells, and thus destroy the virus. Warts which have been unsuccessfully treated using home remedies are generally more difficult to cure than those which have not.

Athlete's foot, a fungal infection of the skin, may be caused by one of a number of fungi *(dermatophytes)*. It is contagious and causes itching of the affected areas. For a definite diagnosis, culture of a scraping in a laboratory is required. The treatment usually consists of at least daily applications of anti-fungal creams, powders or paints by the patient under a chiropodist's or doctor's direction. Athlete's foot is commonly thought to be present when, in fact, the skin is simply too moist.

Other lesions

Ingrown toenails

In this condition the toenail has penetrated the skin, causing a wound, which not infrequently becomes infected. It is usually caused by bad footwear, which pushes the soft flesh onto the edge of the nail, or by bad cutting technique. In virtually all cases some treatment, aimed at removing the offending portion of nail, is required. In early cases, this may not necessitate the use of a local analgesic. In more advanced cases, a variety of techniques may be used, by either chiropodists or surgeons.

Corns and callouses

These are thickenings of normal skin in response to excessive pressure or friction. Both are symptoms of a malfunction between the foot and the shoe. The treatment is both debridement (paring away with a scalpel) of the thickened tissue and, more importantly, diagnosis and correction of the cause. This may be a functional problem in the foot itself, or simply be due to inadequate footwear.

This section presents a quick guide to the type of foot problems which may be found. The importance of children's feet cannot be overstated. A child's foot, because it is still growing, is malleable and is thus vulnerable. Deformities created in the early years become the painful and immobilising foot problems of old age. Choosing the right footwear is an essential part of prevention. In the environment of contemporary Britain, shoes and hose will inevitably be a normal part of living. But too frequently, the shoes which protect the feet from passing external injury also do them lifelong internal damage. Everyone should ensure that their shoes – as Florence Nightingale did with her hospitals – 'at least do no harm'. It is not just the welfare of children and pensioners which is at stake, but the future of the footcare services. Given the physiology of the foot, the only long-term strategy for reducing the excess demand for foot treatments is prevention.

Part II

Need: Unknown, Unmeasured, Unmet

7 Expectant mothers: the 'non' priority group

Expectant mothers have long received special attention from the health services as part of the enduring campaign against infant mortality. It is perhaps, therefore, no surprise that pregnant women were made a priority group for NHS chiropody. What is surprising is that they make so little use of the service. Only 0.2% of chiropodists clinical hours are spent with expectant mothers.

Some chiropodists have worried that because of the long waiting lists for chiropody, pregnancy (and therefore eligibility) may have ended before the women receive appointments. Others have argued that pregnant women have few foot problems and hence little need of footcare. The present study set out to test these theories.

The foot problems of all the women of 37 weeks pregnancy who attended the ante natal clinic of the local maternity hospital were investigated during a week picked at random. Interviews and foot examinations were conducted with 35 women in total.

In the interview, carried out through interpreters in some cases, the women were asked if they had any foot trouble. If so, the following facts were checked: whether the problem pre-dated the pregnancy, if it had got worse as time went by, and whether any action had been taken to deal with it. These were measures of felt need.

The examination went on to detect any further problems which the women themselves did not recognise; their potential need. It also enabled the accuracy of the diagnoses offered by the women to be checked.

Conditions reported and detected

Just under half the sample, 16 women, reported trouble with their feet. The examination revealed problems in an additional four women, so, in total, 57% of the group had some foot condition.

Generally the diagnoses offered by the women were accurate but they did not recognise all their existing problems. This reflects the findings by May Clarke (see page 4) that chiropodists identify more problems than the patients themselves. The table below shows the conditions reported and those found by professional examination. Some women had more than one.

Table 7: Conditions reported and unreported by expectant mothers

Condition	Reported	Unreported but found by chiropodist	Total
Swollen feet	8	—	8
Varicose veins	1	1	2
Aching	3	—	3
Corns	2	2	4
Bunions/painful toe/ minor skeletal	2	7	9
Skin condition	1	—	1
Callous	0	1	1
Nail problem	0	2	
			2
Total conditions	17	13	30
	Felt Need	Potential Need	Total Need

Sixteen women reported foot conditions, and, of these, 12 had problems connected with the veins and venous system. This is not surprising as the increased weight, and pressure on the abdominal venous system is at its highest in the later stage of pregnancy.

The other four women who indicated problems had: a skin condition, a corn, a bunion and a painful toe, plus hard skin. None of these women had sought treatment from a chiropodist or any other source.

Amongst those reporting trouble were six who had other conditions, discovered in the examination, beyond those they mentioned. Five had minor skeletal problems, such as curly toes, and two of these had callouses or corns as well. One also had a nail problem. The sixth woman who had reported aching, was found to have varicose veins.

There were four women who reported no trouble but who had conditions which the examining chiropodists detected. None were painful, although all were recognisable simply by looking at the feet.

The point of detailing these conditions is to demonstrate that all the chiropodial problems (as opposed to the circulatory ones) were minor and did not need urgent treatment.

Total chiropodial conditions found and treatments

Excluding the circulatory conditions (which are properly dealt with by the patient's obstetrician or general pratitioner) 11 women, 35% of the sample, had chiropodial problems. Together, they had 16 conditions:

    9 skeletal (bunions, curly toes, etc.)
    5 skin (corns, callouses, etc.)
    2 nail problems

1. Skeletal problems

Curly toes (toes which do not lie straight and flat) may respond to long-term conservative treatment with silicone rubber splints to hold the toes in a corrected position, but bunions are correctable only with surgery. Advice, at least, would benefit these women, since foot comfort could be enhanced by simple measures such as correctly fitting footwear.

2. Skin conditions

Five women were found to have corns or callouses. All would benefit from treatment to remove lesions but, more importantly, advice on self help and prevention could have been given.

3. Nail problems

Two women were found to have a toe nail which was thickened and distorted. Whilst not giving pain, these nails are difficult to cut. Advice on self management of the condition would be useful.

Only three of the 16 chiropodial conditions were reported as painful, none seriously. From this small sample, it would appear that only 5 (15%) of the women would derive immediate benefit from physical treatment by a chiropodist.

Action taken to relieve foot problems reported

None of the women with foot problems had consulted a chiropodist. Where a foot problem was reported, the woman was asked about any action taken to seek advice or treatment, including self help.

Table 8: Action taken to relieve conditions reported

Circulatory problems:	total detected	=	13
Sources of help used:	Hospital doctor	=	3
	General practitioner	=	2
	Self help	=	3
	Unknown	=	5
Chiropodial problems:	total detected	=	16
Sources of help used:	Self help	=	1
	None	=	15
Other problem:	Total detected	=	1
Source of help:	Hospital doctor	=	1

That none of these women, even the ones with corns and callouses, sought chiropody may disappoint some chiropodists. But, at least, it dispenses with one worry: it certainly is not the chiropodial waiting list which is keeping pregnant women from footcare.

Onset of foot conditions

Whilst the true reason for expectant mothers' enjoyment of 'priority group' status is buried in the past, one justification may well have been the belief that the increase in weight and alteration in posture caused by pregnancy might lead to an increase in foot problems. There is also generally increased sensitivity to the health of expectant mothers which is aimed at reducing infant mortality. Free chiropody may have been included simply on the grounds that expectant mothers are entitled to virtually all medical services free of charge, without questioning too closely whether these services are really needed.

Of the total problems found, 13 had existed before the pregnancy; of these three were circulatory, one a skin condition and nine were 'chiropodial'. Those occurring since pregnancy, eight in all, were all circulatory in nature. Thus, in this small sample, it would seem that chiropodial foot conditions, as opposed to circulatory problems, do not start in pregnancy.

Policy conclusions

This study of expectant mothers suggests that they have only a small amount of unmet need for chiropody. Therefore, as a group, pregnant women do not seem to warrant their priority status. On the other hand, they make so little demand on the service that there is no point in changing their status until there is a general reconsideration of the priority group system. What could be done in the meanwhile is to strengthen the notification, through ante-natal clinics, of the availability of chiropody, so that the few expectant mothers who need it do not overlook the opportunity.

More important is an improved provision of information and advice on foot health. Ante-natal clinics are one of the few places where an adult's health is regularly checked and present an ideal opportunity to give guidance on self care. Women take up most of the chiropody services available to elderly people and intervention earlier in their lives may help them to look after their own feet better. It is also the right moment to teach women about the care of children's feet, which is where the real effort in preventive chiropody needs to be expanded. The level of foot health education in the country is so low at present that chiropodists should take better advantage of the opportunity offered by ante-natal clinics.

8 Schoolchildren: tomorrow's foot problems

Children's feet rarely hurt, so, despite their status as a priority group, schoolchildren take up only 2.8% of chiropodists' clinical time. As already mentioned, their feet are relatively soft and mould painlessly under pressure. But the mouldability which lessens discomfort in youth is simultaneously creating the problems of old age. Feet may become irremediably deformed in the early years, restricting their functioning later, and creating vulnerable pressure points. This is a mass social problem. Most elderly people suffer with their feet, and the chiropody services labour under the unending task of relieving their discomfort. It would clearly be more sensible to correct these skeletal/structural deformities just as they begin to develop, in youth. What children need from the footcare services is not treatment for painful feet **now,** but preventive care to stop their feet from becoming painful **later.**

In fact, such a preventive system already exists: the school health service. School children in the district receive an annual medical inspection which includes an examination of the feet. But most referrals to the school's chiropody clinic are for nail problems or infections such as warts, rather than for structural or functional deficiences. It appears as if the screening operation is missing the emergent skeletal deformations which are the foundation for so much foot trouble later. Thus, the study sought to measure the full extent of foot problems in schoolchildren.

Ideally, the authors would like to have conducted foot examinations with a representative selection of schoolchildren of all ages. In technical sampling terms, this is not difficult. But the administrative problems would have been enormous. The process of obtaining written permission from the parents of each of the several hundred children selected would have taken much more time and resources than were available. And conducting the examinations would have involved disruptions to school timetables.

Instead, the foot examinations were carried out together with school nurses as part of their routine hygiene inspections of whole classes at a time, thus providing a large number of pupils quickly, 205 in all. By selecting class visits, children of all ages between three and fourteen were included. But this was not a rigourous representative sample of the school population.

The examination had two parts: first with the shoes on, fastened, and the child standing; second, with the feet bare. This latter part of the examination included the child standing normally and on tip toe, viewed from both front and rear. Active and passive movements of all the principal joints (ankle, subtalar and metatarso-phalangeal) were checked. The recording also included toe deformities, skin lesions, nail problems, hygiene and gait.

The three principal findings were that, of all the school children examined:

71% had shoes which did not fit;
77% had some problem with their feet;
91% had a problem with either shoes or feet.

The shoe problems are detailed in Chapter 20. The results of the foot examination are shown in Table 9.

Foot problem detected

Over 50% of the children had burrowing fifth toes. Of these, just over half had only this problem, suggesting that footwear alone could be the cause. Burrowing toes, which are rotated sideways on the long axis through the metatarsal, may not give trouble until much later in life. Then, however, the effect of the rotation on function, in combination with arthritis, may be one of continuous pain as corns develop or nails become damaged and thick. The remaining children who had burrowing fifth toes also had other problems such as inrolling feet, knock knees, or curly toes. These last – curly toes – are the subject of debate amongst chiropodists and the medical profession.

It is undoubtedly true that many babies are born with curly toes, and also that many straighten as the child grows and walks. Those which do not, may give rise to foot problems in later life. Thus there is a case for trying to straighten toes if curling has not resolved, or preventive measures in terms of hose and footwear education have

Table 9: Summary of foot problems found

Children		% of children	
47	No foot problems	23.0	
19	Restricted movement	9.2	
2	*Metatarsus varus*	0.97	
4	*primus varus*	1.9	Skeletal
10	*Hallux valgus* (bunions)	4.8	problems
61	Burrowing 5th toes (only)	29.7	
54	Burrowing 5th toes and other toe problems	26.3	
21	Other toe deformities only	10.2	
		83.07	
1	Ingrown nails	0.48	Soft tissue
6	Corns	2.9	problems
10	Callouses	6.8	
		10.18	
13	*Verrucae*	6.3	Infections
2	Athlete's foot	0.97	
		7.27	
19	Poor hygiene	9.2	
269	Total	131%	

N = 205 Children

(The total is over 100% as some children had more than one problem)

Table 10: Summary of results of children's feet survey

```
100

      90                                                            91%

                                                                     F
                                                                     O
      80                                              77%            O
                                                                     T

                                                       F             O
      70                                71%            O             R
                                                       O
Percent                                  S             T             S
  of                                     H                           H
                                         O             P             O
Children                                 E             R             E
(N = 205)                                              O
      60                                 P             B             P
                                         R             L             R
                                         O             E             O
      50                                 B             M             B
                                         L             S             L
                                         E                           E
                                         M                           M
      40                                 S                           S


      30


      20


      10        9%

                 N
                 O
                 N
       0         E
```

failed. Correction is attempted by using 'toe dentures' which are moulded from silicone rubber directly on the foot whilst holding the toes in a corrected position. The silicone sets to a firm consistency, is removable for bathing and is quite painless to wear. Whilst the long-term study of such treatment is still in its early stages, clinical evidence shows that, in some cases, correction can be achieved (see Black and Coates, 1981). Muscle imbalance, the relative positions of the insertions of tendons or cramping by hose or shoes are some of the many causes of curly toes. Some curly toes may result from a combination of malfunction at the subtalar joint (the joint allowing the foot to tilt sideways on the leg) and footwear; these may be curable if both causes are removed. The problem is, however to detect the true causes of curly toes, so that cure is not attempted in the child with intrinsic (internal) causes, as disappointment at failure to correct may deter the person from seeking treatment for other foot conditions later in life.

Some 5% of the children had *hallux valgus* (bunions). Most of these also had signs of the commonly occuring associated problems, such as corns, burrowing fifth toes, callouses, etc. The tendency to develop bunions can of course be inherited, but shoes may aid the acquisition of this deformity. Even if deformity cannot be prevented, attention to footwear may reduce the speed at which *hallux valgus* develops and prevent formation of corns and callosities.

The smaller number of soft tissue lesions than of skeletal ones can be divided into two major groups: infections and others.

1. Infections

Foot warts, *verrucae,* were found in 6.3% of the children. These are virus infections of the skin, common in children, less so in adults. Half were being treated by a variety of agencies, including doctors, and parents giving treatment prescribed by a doctor. The other seven were referred by the chiropodist to the school chiropody service. Another 1% had a fungal infection – 'athlete's foot', and were receiving treatment from the family doctor. One of these children had very mobile feet with curly toes and a small ulcer on his ankle and was referred to the chiropodist for a rigorous clinical examination, as these were felt to be of more importance in the long term than the infection.

2. Other lesions

The other lesions were corns, callouses and ingrown toenails. Corns are skin lesions caused by excessive pressure over a bony prominence or joint. Callosities are a thickening of the superficial skin layers in response to friction. Both are symptoms of disharmony between foot and shoe, and may often be cured, at least in children, by attention to footwear.

A total of 7.8% children were showing physical signs of malfunction between the foot and the shoe in which the cause could be found and cured. Corns and callouses do become painful, and some changes in the skin itself can be detected in long-standing cases. The proportion of older people who have corns and callouses is vast, and much time is spent by chiropodists in treating such lesions. Their prevention would not only improve the comfort of the individual but would also lessen future demand on the chiropody service.

One child was found with ingrown toenails. This is a condition where the toenail is actually penetrating the flesh of the toe. Its commonest causes are poor cutting of the nail and trauma, the flesh being pushed onto the nail edge, eg. by footwear, rather than the nail actually growing in. This condition requires treatment to stop the edge of the nail cutting into the flesh and also correction of the nail shape by smoothing its edge to allow healing. In some cases further treatment is required to prevent recurrence. This child had ingrown nails on both sides of both first toes and, whilst admitting that they were rather painful, had not had any treatment for them. He was given an appointment to attend the school chiropody clinic (where the condition was cured). All the soft tissue lesions seen could have been cured.

Hygiene

The standard of hygiene was high, 86.3% children having a 'good' entered against the hygiene question. Hygiene was judged by the cleanliness of the socks and feet, and by the condition of the skin. Many children had been playing bare-foot games or wearing football socks, and allowance was made for these. Some 5.8% had poor hygiene and a further 3.4% had bad hygiene. One child was recorded as having a very dry skin and eight cases had no record made. Hygiene, in terms of foot health, is probably more of a problem after puberty. It is then that odour becomes a particular problem.

There is, however, a small but real need for children and parents to understand the importance of foot hygiene. The shoe – a warm, dark and enclosing structure – provides bacteria and fungi with the ideal conditions for growth, along with moisture from the foot. A damp skin will, if not cared for, peel away, especially between the toes, leaving a breach in the body's defences against infections. A very dry skin may also crack open causing pain and allowing infection at entry point. Dry skins also need care, in the form of creams or lotion, to increase the suppleness of the skin.

Hygiene is obviously a subject about which school nurses know a good deal and it should not be difficult to equip them with specialist knowledge on foot hygiene.

Responses to the problem

Curly toes, the most common finding, and especially the burrowing fifth toes, whilst painless in childhood, may give acute pain in later life as their function is impaired. In elderly people the treatment of such toes takes up much of the chiropodists' time, and it has already been shown that the majority of NHS chiropody is devoted to elderly people (85.9%). This costly way of dealing with foot problems could be avoided if there were a preventive and corrective service to children. A service which is palliative after the damage has been done is self limiting in terms of the number of patients to whom foot comfort can be given, as each patient will need regular chiropody for life. Whilst surgery may well provide a cure, orthopaedic surgeons almost always have waiting lists and many more urgent operations. Also, many older people do not want, or are not fit enough to undergo surgery unless it is life saving.

If there is to be any hope of providing everyone with foot comfort there must be a policy to correct 'minor' problems in childhood so that the proportion of old people with foot trouble is dimished.

Many of the conditions found were within the scope of a chiropodist, none were being treated by one. Some children were receiving treatment from the doctor.

The overall picture then was of a very large number of children with unmet potential need for foot treatments of various kinds. The implication is that current screening methods are failing to detect the vast majority of foot problems in children, even though the feet are being inspected, and 88% of these children are likely to have foot problems when they reach pensionable age.

There are various responses to the problem: it may be argued that many of the problems correct themselves spontaneously, so the current policy of doing little is the correct one, or alternatively, that all children should be screened by a chiropodist, which is impractical in the existing manpower shortage.

A third option may prove both practical and cost-effective, without any loss in terms of effectiveness. The school nurses, already conducting annual hygiene inspections, could, with some extra training detect the skeletal and functional problems which should be referred to a chiropodist for further investigation, advice or treatment. The detection of skin lesions would continue, and, if the inspection were expanded to include footwear, the screening would become even more effective. There is a distinct need for education and advice on footwear as well as on feet, which school nurses could give, provided they had sufficient knowledge.

The district studied has chosen this third option. It is planning to organise a training workshop to help school nurses increase the detection of skeletal and footwear problems, as well as the currently detected skin lesions. The nurses themselves have expressed enthusiasm for the project.

It is early days yet, but the prospect for a substantial increase in preventive work with the young for virtually no increased expenditure is both exciting and possible.

9 Research method: interview, examination, recommendation

The distinction between two methods of investigating foot problems has already been pointed out: to ask people about their foot troubles and for a professionally trained person to conduct a clinical examination. Both are important. The self-report is a measure of 'felt need'. The clinical examination identifies the full 'potential need'.

People often fail to recognise their foot problems until advancing age renders them painful as well as more serious. By the time that they are brought to the attention of the footcare services, they are often difficult to deal with by anything other than temporary, pain-relieving treatment. So, if preventive footcare is to be developed, problems must be caught as they are just emerging by conducting foot examinations as well as asking people about their problems.

This combination is the method used in all the present studies of unmet need and also in the investigation of the service currently provided by chiropody. In the two studies already reported, especially the school children, the conditions under which the research was conducted meant that the interview had to be briefer and less formal. In four other studies (of handicapped people, elderly people, and those on the waiting list, plus the chiropody service itself) more thorough and rigorous interviews with all patients were conducted. The questions covered their degree of mobility, their medical history, their present physical condition relevant to foot health, their footwear and their attitudes towards it, their recognition of their own foot problems, and how they dealt with them, including any previous use of chiropody.

Clinical foot examinations of all patients were carried out by state registered chiropodists. For the large study of the chiropody service, every member of the department's staff took part in the examinations. In all cases, the chiropodists recorded the problems present on a long list of foot conditions and recommended the form of footcare appropriate to the patient from a list of ten options ranging over advice, routine treatment, intensive treatment, footcare assistance, discharge. This choice was clearly designed to be an 'ideal' one. At the time of the research, not all the options were available within the district's chiropody service. For example, no footcare assistant was then in post. The purpose of structuring the recommendations in this way was, in part, to measure the difference between the theoretically best forms of treatment and the services the department was actually delivering. This gap is simultaneously a rough measure of inappropriate care for the patient and inefficiency in the chiropody service.

The ten treatment options are shown in Table 11. When the results of these studies were analysed the various treatment plans which the individual patients received were first totalled. Then, to see what pattern of service these recommendations implied for the chiropody department as a whole, the treatment plans were grouped into five patterns of care – *minimal treatment* (care that involves only a small amount of work for the service), *curative treatment* (where the patient is successfully discharged), *occasional treatment* (which implies continuing relationships with the patients, but only on an infrequent basis), *footcare assistance* (where the long-term care necessary can be given by a footcare assistant), and *chiropody for life* (where the patients will require frequent, routine treatments for the rest of their lives). From the Table, it can be seen that many of these long-term patterns of care depend on an initial course of intensive treatment to bring the patient's feet up to the best possible condition. Five of the treatment plans involve this intensive treatment at the outset: numbers four, five, six, eight and nine. This is a particularly important form of care, costly in the short-term, economical in the long run, so separate analysis was carried out of the number of times intensive treatment was recommended for patients.

With small variations in the questions, this same combination of interview, foot examination and treatment recommendation was used in all four of the studies mentioned. It took the form of a six-page schedule for each patient (see Appendix I). However, the means by which the appropriate people were located varied between the four studies, with handicapped people presenting a particularly interesting problem. The details of how patients were selected and how the physical process of research was organised is described in the individual chapters. Amidst the details, however, one must not forget the overall purpose: to locate unmet need in the patients and inefficiency in the provision of service.

Table 11: Chiropody treatment plans and patterns of footcare

These *treatment plans* —————— imply —————— these *patterns of care*

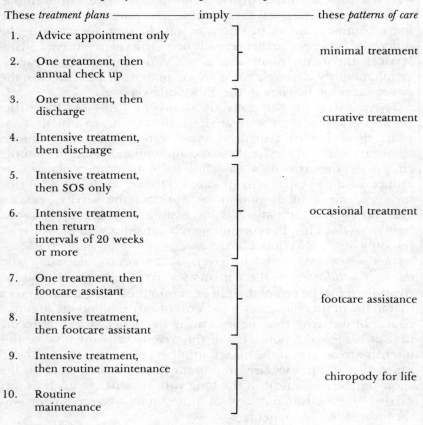

1. Advice appointment only	
	minimal treatment
2. One treatment, then annual check up	
3. One treatment, then discharge	
	curative treatment
4. Intensive treatment, then discharge	
5. Intensive treatment, then SOS only	
	occasional treatment
6. Intensive treatment, then return intervals of 20 weeks or more	
7. One treatment, then footcare assistant	
	footcare assistance
8. Intensive treatment, then footcare assistant	
9. Intensive treatment, then routine maintenance	
	chiropody for life
10. Routine maintenance	

10 Handicapped people: in despair of care

Not all handicapped people have problems adequately represented by that now accepted symbol, the wheelchair. But many suffer from restricted mobility, so it is important to maintain whatever freedom of movement they have. That is the logic behind giving handicapped people priority access to chiropody. Their footcare needs will vary, in part, with their physical condition. For visually handicapped but able bodied people, the requirement may simply be for a toenail-cutting service. Others may need more extensive treatment, including orthotics (insoles, etc) to aid their comfort and mobility.

It is characteristic of handicapped people that they do not claim all the benefits to which they are legally entitled, and this applies to their use of chiropody services. In Warren's study, mentioned in the introduction (see page 4), some 30% of handicapped people felt they needed footcare, but only 14% were receiving it. The national survey by Harris, Cox and Smith roughly confirmed this level of use, with 17% receiving chiropody. Certainly, the amount of time chiropodists spend treating handicapped people, only 4.2% of their clinical hours, seems surprisingly low. Thus, there is reason to suspect substantial levels of unmet need.

One of the consequences of this renunciation of legal entitlements is that people who would like to assess their needs have difficulty in finding them. The local Registers of Disabled Persons are known to cover only about 60% of those eligible. There were no resources to follow Warren's example and make a complete census of the research district.

Fortunately, one of the adjacent London boroughs does have an accurate list of handicapped people within part of its geographical area. This borough had a low-lying region at risk from inundation

until the new Thames flood defences were completed. An annual
door-knocking exercise located the handicapped people who could
not escape unaided. The list included, as well as name and address,
details of age and handicap. The compilation also used a very
precise and relevant definition of 'handicapped people' – 'those
who could not remove to a place of safety (from a flood zone)
without help'. The list only covers a small geographical area, but is
complete within these limits. This was basis for the present
research.

Two hundred and five people were listed, one of whom was
excluded from the study because he had a bilateral leg amputation.
Cross-checking with the chiropody service's master index for the
area determined that exactly 25% of handicapped people (51 of 204)
were already receiving NHS chiropody treatment. This is a higher
level of use than found in the other studies, perhaps a result of the
borough's determined effort to locate handicapped people in this
small area.

At the same time, this means that 75% were not in contact with the
footcare services. To see if any unmet need existed in this group, a
20% sample was taken; all the selected people were asked by letter if
they would consent to an inteview and foot examination in their
own homes; in the end, 16 useable interviews were completed.
These represent just over 10% of the people who are not already
receiving chiropody.

The people studied did indeed suffer from restricted mobility.
Less than a fifth could leave their homes alone and only two could
use a bus. All of the sixteen, however, could be brought to a clinic in
a tail-lift vehicle.

Only three of the people studied were under retirement age, so
that 13 were eligible for chiropody on grounds of being elderly as
well as being handicapped. They had double priority for treatment.

Their range of handicap is particularly relevant to footcare. There
were five whose principal handicap was arthritis of one sort or
another; three had strokes, two bronchitis, two heart conditions,
one low blood pressure, one multiple sclerosis and one an
unidentified psychiatric illness. The majority of these conditions
affected the way in which foot treatment must be given. These are
the kinds of medical complications mentioned earlier, which mean
that even simple footcare must be delivered by a skilled
professional.

In the opinion of the examining chiropodist, ten of the 16 patients, 62%, required chiropody treatment. This is a measure of unmet need. Three others would have benefitted from advice and for another an annual check-up was a desirable precaution. The ten who needed treatment had 20 foot conditions in all. Relatively few of these were corns and callouses, which are caused by pressure and friction on the skin. The handicapped person's restricted mobility may reduce these particular problems. The full list of conditions discovered is shown in Table 12.

Table 12: Foot conditions in handicapped people (unmet need)

Nail cutting only	5
Bunions	5
Callouses	5
Lesser toe deformities	4
Corns	1
TOTAL	20

In terms of the physical treatments required, these unmet needs of handicapped people were simple. But they did require care, both for comfort and mobility. However, none of these patients could be safely treated by a footcare assistant, relative or amateur volunteer. Their medical condition puts them at greater risk from infection or ulcerations. All ten required care by a chiropodist.

Among handicapped people in this area a quarter were already receiving chiropody. Of the remaining three-quarters, some 62% of the sample had minor foot conditions that required professional attention, suggesting that over 70% needed footcare in some degree of whom most were not receiving any. These are much higher estimates of need than in previous research.

Policies for the future

Of course, the present investigation of unmet need was a very small one, indeed the smallest of all the ten studies. Part of the explanation of the much higher figure may lie in the size of the sample. Part also certainly lies in the fact that the present study was the only one of handicapped people which involved a clinical foot examination. The authors would not want to draw any firm conclusions from such limited evidence. The volume of need which the study suggests, however, is sufficiently large to deserve further investigation on a large scale, all the more because even the relatively simple unmet needs of handicapped people could become dangerous if treated inappropriately.

Immediate action is possible, however, on one additional sad finding of research. Seven of the patients recognised that they had a foot problem of some sort. None had applied for chiropody treatment. When asked why, five of them said they did not think treatment was available. They knew they could be helped by a chiropodist and that such a service exists, but felt that they could not get access to it.

This represents a disturbing failure of communication. Most of the people studied, in fact, had double priority for chiropody. Many must have social workers who visit them and should advise on the services available. The voluntary organisations concerned with handicapped people have been increasingly active in recent years, especially in the area of providing information services. Yet many handicapped people in need of footcare still do not know they are eligible. The straightforward job of education to be done here could best be undertaken by the statutory and voluntary agencies who are already in contact with handicapped people.

In addition, voluntary and statutory agencies could help by providing transport as, in a given period of time, chiropodists can treat approximately twice the number of patients in a clinic as in home visits.

One task which should not be undertaken, however, is voluntary toenail cutting, as the medical conditions of handicapped people often mean that even simple footcare cannot always be safely dealt with by untrained personnel. The commitment which is needed from all agencies, however, is to fund and help organise a major investigation into the footcare needs of handicapped people. The research suggests that they are larger than anyone previously suspected.

11 Elderly people: the measurement of stoicism

Elderly people are the largest consumers of National Health Service chiropody services, receiving over 20 times as much as the next largest patient group (Table 6). Nonetheless, almost every survey which asks elderly people about services which they need or want, produces requests for more chiropody, usually at or near the top of the list.

Chiropodists themselves acknowledge the solid basis for this demand. By the Chief Chiropody Officers' own estimate, the NHS has less than half the chiropodists it needs to treat elderly people adequately. Thus, we have good reason to believe that despite their already large call on services, there is substantial unmet need for footcare among the pension-age population.

For this most important group of patients, therefore, the authors wanted to assess need in all its many forms, as described earlier in Chapter 2. That meant, for a start, determining what portion of the elderly population is already in receipt of public or private footcare services, that is, 'met need' or current provision. Then come the various grades of unmet need. First, there are people who have activated requests for service, but have not yet received it, those on the waiting list for chiropody. Second, others know they have foot problems but for some reason have not sought help, what is called 'felt need'. Third, there are the foot problems revealed by a clinical examination but of which people themselves are not aware, 'potential need'. Further, they wanted to assess how serious these unmet needs were and what treatments the conditions required; that is, they wanted to translate these unmet needs into requirements for various types of care. Then, by combining those already receiving services with those in unmet need they wanted to produce an estimate of the total need for footcare amongst elderly people.

Finally and happily, there is also a group which has no need of treatment.

Ideally, the authors would like to have conducted a general survey of elderly people in the community. But many technical problems are involved in organising such a study and, in any case, it was well beyond the available resources. As a surrogate, many people who have studied elderly people, like Townsend and Wedderburn (see Appendix II), have used general practitioners' lists as a means of drawing a sample. Most people are registered with a doctor, so the patient lists of all the GPs in an area provide reasonably complete coverage of the population. This approach was tried. In principle, the local Family Practitioner Committee was willing to help, but there were administrative problems which would have delayed the fieldwork beyond the time available. So, instead, a complete census of all the old people attending a large local health centre during a week picked at random was conducted. There are two potential biases in this method, working in opposite directions. Most people who come to the doctor are in some sense 'sick' and hence perhaps more likely to have yet other health problems (including foot problems) than the rest of the population. On the other hand, unlike many elderly people, these attenders are at least in contact with the health services and hence more likely to have had their problems dealt with than others. While these difficulties cannot be ignored, the study revealed a volume of need for footcare so massive as to swamp any technical biases in research method.

All the elderly people who came to the health centre were met during their visit. The research study was explained and they were asked if they would participate. Of the 90 who attended that week, six declined. Another 13 agreed in principle but were unable to take part for a variety of practical reasons.

The 71 who formed the study were asked if they were currently receiving footcare from any source. There were 31 attending NHS chiropody clinics. A further five reported having regular care from a private chiropodist or pedicurist. No other sources of professional help were mentioned. No interview-examination with these 36 people was conducted, because a much larger study of those currently having chiropody had been done, (see Chapter 17). The point here is that just over 50% of elderly people were already receiving some form of footcare service.

All the remaining people were asked if they were waiting for any footcare services. Three people reported being on the waiting list for NHS chiropody. This 4.2% (3/71) is about what one would expect. Some four and a half per cent of the elderly population of the district was on the waiting list for chiropody at the time. No one mentioned waiting for any other footcare services. Again, the interview-examination was not conducted, because a thorough study of the waiting list had already been done (see Chapter 12).

After deducting those already receiving or waiting for treatment, 32 people, some 45%, were not in contact with any footcare services. This is the group the authors wanted to study intensively and which participated in the interview-examination. In this group, which had heretofore shown no need for help, 59% of the people (19 out of 32) reported trouble with their feet. This is a measure of 'felt need'. Some reported more than one condition. And the foot examination confirmed that they all had the problems which they claimed – plus a few more which they did not. The difficulties they mentioned are set out in Table 13.

Table 13: Conditions reported by elderly people NOT receiving footcare (felt need)

Corns	7
Nail problems	5
Pain	4
Callouses	3
Infection	1
Hot feet	1
'Strange' sensation	1
Unrecorded	1
	23

N = 19 people, three people reporting more than one condition.

All these conditions could have been dealt with by a chiropodist. In some cases, it might have been necessary to refer the patient to a doctor for investigations of circulation or other systemic conditions. In others, help from a footcare assistant would have been sufficient.

Why did these people who reported foot trouble not seek treatment? One woman admitted that she was too frightened to go to a chiropodist. A man in a generally poor state of health acknowledged he had been neglecting himself. Both recognised that a chiropodist could help. In contrast, two others felt they could manage to treat themselves. But 14 people, in one way or another, avoided answering the question, a common and revealing response in this context.

People often avoid acting on their problems. Many expect their feet to deteriorate and become painful as a natural part of ageing. They see the problem as inevitable and irremediable.

Health education is obviously needed here. People must realise that, while foot trouble is common, it does not have to be tolerated or accepted as part of growing old. As was pointed out, it may be impossible to undo long-standing skeletal deformity, but much can be done to improve foot function and/or comfort. People can be helped through teaching them more about basic footcare and the proper choices of footwear. Chiropodists will never be able to do this education job alone. Old people's clubs, social workers, district nurses and voluntary groups working with elderly people could all play a part in disseminating information.

Foot examination

After the interview, a chiropodist conducted the foot examination. Among the 13 patients who reported no trouble, the chiropodists discovered three people needing treatment and two others who would soon have problems unless they received footwear advice. This is one indicator of 'potential need'. But there was also another. In six of the 19 people who reported foot trouble, the examining chiropodists identified other conditions which the patients themselves had not recognised. Again, all could have been dealt with by chiropody.

Table 14: Unreported foot problems (potential need)

Corns	4
Nails	3
Fungal infection	2
Callous	2
Footwear	2
TOTAL	13

The types of foot troubles which people overlook are of interest. Putting the two groups with potential need together, including two people who had two conditions each, there were 13 problems.

For all those 24 patients where the interview-examination revealed some unmet need (that is, the 19 who reported conditions plus the additional five where problems were found during the foot examination), the chiropodists recommended the course of action they felt would be most suitable if people were to be given treatment. Their recommendations are analysed in Table 15.

Table 15: Treatment required by elderly people with unmet needs

Treatment recommendation	Problem reported (Felt Need) N = 19	Problem discovered (Potential Need) N = 5	All problems N = 24	Pattern of care	
Plan No:					
1. Advice only	16.7	8.3	25.0	33.3	Minimal treatment
2. 1 treatment annually	8.3	—	8.3		
3. 1 treatment, discharge	—	—	—	0.0	Curative treatment
4. Intensive treatment then discharge	—	—	—		
5. Intensive treatment then SOS	25.0	8.3	33.3	37.5	Occasional treatment
6. Intensive treatment then long intervals	4.2	—	4.2		
7. 1 treatment only then foot-care asst.	12.5	4.2	16.7	20.9	Footcare assistance
8. Intensive treatment then FCA	4.2	—	4.2		
9. Intensive treatment then routine maintenance	8.3	—	8.3	8.3	Chiropody for life
10. Routine maintenance	—	—	—		
TOTALS	79.2%	20.8%	100%	100%	

These recommendations could be interpreted in two very different ways. An optimist might suggest that the unmet needs of elderly people were rather mild. Over 70% of the recommendations were for only minimal or occasional treatment. And of those who required long-term help, over two thirds only required footcare assistants. The pessimist would observe that half the patients needed intensive treatment before they could be stabilised on these modest levels of care. That is, if all those recommendations which indicate that intensive treatment is needed are combined (numbers four, five, six, eight and nine), it is found that this is appropriate for exactly 50% of the cases. From the perspective of the patient, pessimism is appropriate. Remember that people who have never asked for footcare in any form are being considered here. Yet most of them (almost 80%) know they have a problem, and for 50% a course of intensive treatment is the recommendation. These are measures of stoicism in elderly people. Such self abnegation deserves a compassionate response. More concretely, it deserves footcare.

Table 16: Total footcare needs of elderly people

RECEIVING TREATMENT		50.7%
NHS Chiropody	31 (43.7%)	
Private footcare	5 (7.0%)	
SUB-TOTAL	36 (50.7%)	
UNMET NEED		38.0%
Activated (on waiting list)	3 (4.2%)	
Felt (reported by patient)	19 (26.8%)	
Potential (discovered by chiropodist)	5 (7.0%)	
	27 (38.0%)	
NO NEED	8 (11.3%)	11.3%
TOTAL	71 (100%)	100.0%

The final category in the study of elderly people must now be considered. At the beginning there were 71 patients, 36 of whom were receiving treatment. The three forms of unmet need (waiting list, felt need, potential need), accounted for 27 more. In total then, 63 were in need of help, virtually all of which could be provided by chiropodists. This leaves a residual group of eight people. These are people with healthy feet. That is to say, only 11.3% of elderly people have no need of footcare.

All the findings can now be brought together in a composite table of the footcare needs of the elderly people (see Table 16).

In total, 88.7% of elderly people need some form of footcare. This is a higher estimate than in any previous research. It is almost treble Townsend and Wedderburn's estimate of 30% (1965) and more than half again as high as Clarke's 50% (1969). Even if the small number of patients (six) who needed advice only are eliminated from the figures, the total need is still over 80%. From these figures we can understand why elderly people are requesting ever more chiropody. They imply that the shortage of chiropodists is even more acute than previously thought. And the demographic swell in the elderly population is only just beginning.

This was a small study, conducted by less than ideal methods. But the differences from previous studies are sufficiently great to warrant replication of the research on a larger and more rigorous basis. The levels of need it revealed are also sufficiently alarming to warrant the provision of footcare on a larger and more comprehensive basis.

12 Waiting list: the visible end of the queue

The very idea of a waiting list implies passivity. But those who sit and wait for chiropody are, in another sense, the active ones. Many of the people discovered to have substantial unmet needs for footcare in various social groups recognised they had a foot problem, but had done nothing about it (felt need). Others did not recognise they even had a problem (potential need). But those on the waiting list had both recognised their trouble and done something appropriate about it; they had applied for chiropody. This is what was earlier called 'activated need'. But while they waited their footcare needs were still not being met; indeed, they were probably getting worse.

At the time of the research it took about a year to get to the top of the district's chiropody waiting list. This is a long time to wait when one has something as painful as a corn; it is a long time to get something done as simple as thinning a thick nail. But in other parts of the country, the waiting time can last anything up to five years. To understand how such long waiting lists can come about, one must understand the structural situation in which the NHS chiropody services have become locked.

Under the priority group system, almost nine-tenths of the patients are elderly. Most of their foot problems are by that stage incurable and all that can be done for them is temporary, pain-relieving treatment. But if this palliation is really to control their discomfort it must be repeated frequently for the rest of their lives. Thus, once having got to the chiropody department, most patients become regular visitors, and never leave again for any length of time.

Faced with such an imbalanced selection of patients, there are only five ways in which vacancies are created, none of them easy.

1. Employment of another chiropodist. This would mean another 400 patients could be taken on. But if the chiropodial manpower shortage doesn't block this solution, the public expenditure cuts will.

2. The patient moves out of the district. Elderly people move seldom and in any case this solution is out of the chiropody service's control.

3. The patient dies. This is also beyond the service's management, but because so many of the people are of advanced age, this is, in fact, the most common reason patients cease receiving chiropody.

4. Lengthening the interval between treatments. If existing patients are seen less, one can create vacancies for new patients. But this might mean giving people less than the appropriate treatment for their problems.

5. Discharging patients. Because so many of the foot conditions of elderly people stem from underlying skeletal deformities, it is seldom possible to cure and discharge them. One could, of course, discharge them without curing them first, but that is hardly the solution to the problem of the waiting list one wants.

None of these five options occurs frequently, so few appointments fall vacant. The waiting list moves only slowly.

The waiting list in the district at the time of the research was 849 people, approximately four and a half per cent of the pension-age population of the area. This was all that was known before the research began. An application form was available for each individual. This, the only format in which requests for service are accepted, can be obtained from clinics, home help offices, GP surgeries, social services departments' offices and from the chiropody office itself.

Forms may be submitted by the applicants or anyone else on their behalf. The result is that a large number of them are incompletely filled out and do not form a useable record of the waiting list. The clerks who screen, sort and file the applications in chronological order had the feeling that most of the people were elderly and female. It was necessary to discover the needs of the people who waited: how many had severe problems needing urgent attention, how many could be dealt with quickly and discharged, how many were trivial requests for foot hygiene rather than chiropody, and how many were going to become patients of the department for the rest of their lives.

Starting with the applicants who had been waiting the longest, people from the waiting list were sent appointments to come to the clinic nearest their home for an interview and foot examination. Some 62% of the total list were sent for, and a total of 394 (46%) people actually attended during the time available for the field-work. All had been waiting for periods between 12 and 6 months.

At the appointment no treatment was offered, but details were recorded of the person's mobility, medical history and treatment along with details of previous footcare treatments (if any) and footwear. A clinical examination followed, along with an assessment of the urgency of the person's need, and a recommendation of the optimum treatment plan, when such treatment could be implemented. This effectively divided the waiting list into two major sections: urgent and non-urgent, each of these being subdivided by the type of intervention which was required. Thus, whilst the waiting list would still exist, it would be a list sorted by need, rather than by chronology.

The study, whilst designed to provide factual information about the unmet needs of the waiting list proved so useful as a review/screening mechanism that the system set up for the research continued after the fieldwork time expired, and, with some minor modifications, is still operating. This means that people who apply now have their needs assessed within a few weeks of application.

Age/sex analysis

The analysis of the sex and age of the 394 people confirmed the suppositions of the clerical staff who deal with the application forms when they arrive at the office.

67.5% were women and 32.5% men. The ages ranged from 29 years to 97 years but there were only ten women below retiring age (60) and only three men below 65. Thus the overwhelming majority of those on the waiting list were elderly, one sixth being over 80 years of age.

Urgency results

The screening of application forms is done by a chiropodist who reads all the forms, looking at details given of the foot problem and medical history or treatment in order to give priority to any applicants who have urgent conditions. These include ulcers or sepsis, and medical conditions which put them at risk, such as diabetes or rheumatoid arthritis. In theory then there should not be any 'urgent' cases on the waiting list.

After the interview/examination the chiropodist was asked to decide on the degree of urgency with which the person required treatment. The choices offered were:

1. discharge completely;
2. annual check up only;
3. return to waiting list for treatment;
4. urgently in need of treatment.

Of these, 31.9% were noted as urgent whilst 65.6% could be returned to the waiting list. Thus, in a list which theoretically contains no urgent cases, almost a third were considered to be in urgent need.

The reasons for this may include:

1. lack of information on the referral form which leads to a wrong decision by the chiropodist reading the form, or

2. the length of the wait which allows urgency to develop, for example an untreated nail pressing on to footwear may eventually cause the underlying tissue to break down, giving rise to an ulcer.

Both situations are impossible to prevent completely, but both could be made less likely by an improvement in the design of the referral form and by an assessment/examination at the time of application.

There were only six people in the study who could be discharged immediately. It would seem then that people do not apply for chiropody treatment unless they actually need some form of footcare. Whether they need chiropody or foot hygiene will be illustrated by the treatment plans chosen by the chiropodists.

Treatment plans

A treatment plan was indicated in 378 cases, and all ten options were used. The distribution of the people is shown in Table 17.

Table 17: Treatment plans for those on the waiting list

1. Advice appointment only	1.3		
		4.5	minimal treatment
2. One treatment, then annual check up	3.2		
3. One treatment, then discharge	1.6		
		5.5	curative treatment
4. Intensive treatment, then discharge	3.9		
5. Intensive treatment, then SOS only	7.6		
		21.6	occasional treatment
6. Intensive treatment, then return intervals of 20 weeks or more	14.0		
7. One treatment, then footcare assistant	14.5		
		22.1	footcare assistance
8. Intensive treatment, then footcare assistant	7.6		
9. Intensive treatment, then routine maintenance	15.3		
		45.9	chiropody for life
10. Routine maintenance	30.6		
	99.6%		

For nearly one third of the list, the chosen option was routine maintenance, which effectively means chiropody for life. This will, of course, add to the problem of blocking of appointments once they have gained access to the system. In fact, the situation is made worse when those people who need routine maintenance after a course of intensive treatment (plan 9) are added in – a further 15.3%, bringing the total to 45.9%.

Of the waiting list, 14.5% were considered suitable for footcare after an initial chiropody treatment. A further 7.6% were considered to need intensive chiropody before being transferred to footcare appointments. Thus, by the employment of an FCA, some 22.1% of those on the waiting list, could, over a short period of time, receive the footcare they require.

Intensive treatment plans were considered appropriate in over one third of cases. At the time of the fieldwork this was not a popular innovation, as it meant a reduction in the routine clinics. The immediate effect was that some people had to wait a little longer for their treatment. The appointments system was flexible enough to allow patients to attend at frequent intervals without any additional clerical work.

Some patients needing intensive care could not then be discharged, although they would not need to be seen routinely. They would, at some time, require further intensive treatment, such as a new orthotic, or a toe nail thinned. For these, an SOS system was devised. A card is given to the patient when the course of treatment is finished. They return it to the chiropody office when they feel they need treatment again and it is guaranteed that they will receive an appointment with 1 to 3 weeks of re-application, depending on the reason for the request. This course of action was appropriate for 7.6% of the waiting list.

4.5% could be discharged after either advice or one treatment. In addition another 5.5% needed curative treatment. But the major problem with such an approach was found to be people's fears that 'discharge' would mean that they would have to wait another 6 to 12 months before being seen again. The patient naturally resists such a course of action, even if the chiropodist feels it to be appropriate. They too were given SOS cards.

The SOS system is increasingly used for people who are discharged as this allows them quick and easy access if they feel they need to come for treatment again. Therefore, some 17.6% of the waiting list are able to have treatment but are not regular attenders, and thus do not contribute to the 'blocking' of appointments. The people on the waiting list thus display varying degrees of urgency of need, and a variety of types of need. Having looked at these two major points of interest, attention was turned to the methods by which people found out about, and applied for, the service. The aim was to discover if they received help with their feet from any source whilst they waited.

Method of application

For each patient there was a referral form or letter, and in 275 cases it was possible to identify the person who had submitted the application. This gave an idea of where most referrals classed as non-urgent came from. (Urgent cases are seen immediately and referrals are filed with patient's records.) As might be expected, 228 (or 82.9%) of the 275 people had completed the forms themselves. Only five had been referred by relatives or neighbours. The remaining 42 cases were referred by doctors, social services, district nurses or health visitors. This low proportion of 'professional' referrals may be accounted for by the fact that their referral forms contain more medical information, and may thus be more often considered urgent. This is not, however, the full story, as people were also asked how they found out how to apply.

Whilst most forms were actually completed by the applicant, the ways in which people found out about the service were more varied. In addition to the 70 who learned of it from their doctor, another 59 either knew or found out how to apply themselves. Friends told 53 people how to apply, and neighbours another 17 people. Relatives also played a much greater part in telling people how to apply, 36, as opposed to only two who actually completed the form for them. Social services (10) district nurses (20) and chiropodists (10) also gave information enabling people to apply for treatment for themselves. Of the 70 people who said that they found out through their doctor, only 15 were actually referred by the doctor completing a form or writing a letter. Most, 51, filled in the form themselves, one was completed by a district nurse, the other three were completed by relatives or neighbours. This would suggest that most doctors expect patients to fill in forms themselves, or perhaps only personally refer patients whom they consider to be in most need. It is certain that doctors do not actually write as many referrals as they orally suggest ought to receive chiropody. Patients are thus sometimes referred by the doctor but this is not apparent because the patient completes the application. This may be important: the two forms were different in design and colour and clerks may have attached more importance to 'professional' referrals. The chiropodists who did the checking should not have been so influenced, but it is possible that they were. A new form has therefore been designed for everyone to complete, as patients are usually capable of recording the conditions for which they take pills, tablets or medicine, even if they cannot name the drug. This is especially true if they take the form home with them to complete.

Other source of help

As none of the patients were receiving treatment from the NHS, it was necessary to find out whether they had ever had treatment from other chiropodists or pedicurists.

Over half (220) had never had any private treatment of any sort for their feet. In 40 of these cases the chiropodist conducting the examination considered the person in urgent need. Of the remainder, 27 had attended a private pedicurist, 96 a private chiropodist, 23 had received NHS chiropody at some time in the past, and 11 had tried a variety of sources of treatment.

Thus it would appear that at least 39% of the people on the waiting list had received care at some time for their feet from someone other than a relative, friend or themselves.

However, when the patients were asked about current usage of services a very different pattern emerged. Only 47 (11.9%) were currently receiving help from anyone other than a relative. The district nurses were cutting nails for 5 people, 14 were attending pedicurists and 28 were going to a private chiropodist.

Thus, very few people receive any footcare whilst on the NHS chiropody waiting list. When it is remembered that a third of these people need urgent treatment and that altogether 60% will need at least regular footcare assistance or chiropody for life, this is strong indication of real unmet need amongst elderly people.

Nail cutting

Most adults take this task for granted, and readers who are not chiropodists or in contact with elderly people may not realise that nail cutting is such a severe and widespread problem. Inability to have one's toenails cut can be the cause of much misery and, because it is thought to be such a simple, routine activity, a source of shame for those who cannot manage it.

In the survey patients were asked if they could cut their own nails, or if not, who did it for them. The chiropodist also noted if it was safe for the nail cutter to continue. Nails cut badly can be worse than nails not cut at all, and the degree of safety was judged by inspecting the nails during the clinical examination.

Only 154 (39.0%) could cut their own nails or get it done safely by someone else. This means that for 240 (61.0%) of the waiting list, their toenails were cut badly. This can have serious consequences. Badly cut but otherwise normal nails may be a cause of ingrown toenails where the nail penetrates the skin, giving an open wound. This may lead to infection, which in old people whose circulation is not so good, may be far more serious in its effects, and more difficult to cure. Thickened or very brittle nails are often found in older people and if these are not cut and thinned, the pressure from footwear can be acute. This is especially true if the nail has lost its normal curvature when viewed from the tip of the toe.

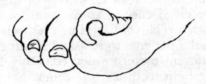

Fig. 3: Nail thickened and with increased curvature

Caught between the bone and the nail, both of which are rigid, the flesh may collapse under the excess pressure, forming an ulcer. This too can become infected. Whilst people whose nails have already caused these conditions will be treated urgently and will not knowingly be put on the waiting list, it is probable that many of the 44.2% who cannot have their nails cut safely will develop these conditions during the year they spend on the waiting list and thus will be urgent cases by the time they are seen at a chiropody clinic. That is obviously the worst possible way of dealing with the problem. Prevention is both less painful and less time consuming and therefore less costly.

Waiting list policy

The waiting list represents therefore a genuine need for footcare, of all types. The policy changes required are those which would, at least, prevent people with urgent needs being missed at the initial filtering stage. This is almost impossible unless every applicant is interviewed and examined at the time of application. As this is impractical, a two-stage strategy has been adopted in the research district. The forms are still scanned on arrival by a chiropodist, and those obviously urgent given an appointment. The rest are sorted by geographic location and filed chronologically. As soon as there are ten applications for any given clinic (or four weeks has elapsed) appointments are sent for an assessment session. This is based on the schedule used in this study, but has undergone some minor adjustments to simplify the computerisation of patients' appointments. No treatment is given, but time is taken to explain the nature of the foot problems and footwear, the proposed plan of treatment, including, where applicable, the fact that they will not get chiropody for life.

This assessment serves a variety of purposes, one of which is to catch the 'urgent' cases which were not obvious from the application. Additionally it allows detection of cases where the need is only for foot hygiene, or a short course of chiropody followed by foot hygiene appointments. People who need only advice or check-ups are also removed from the waiting list at this stage, as are those with conditions which can be cured and the patient 'discharged', such as one thick nail which can be dealt with by avulsion (removal) with destruction of the growth area.

The waiting list remaining thus now consists of people for whom long-term, palliative treatment is going to be the answer. They may still be in considerable discomfort, however, and since the subsequent wait can be considerable they may develop an urgent condition during this period. To deal with these, and many other people who demand treatment instantly, an emergency chiropody clinic has been started. Anyone may attend, on any week day, providing that he or she arrives before a specified time. Only the condition causing pain is treated and the person returned to the waiting list, given a return appointment or discharged as appropriate. The service has proved almost too popular, which imposes a strain on the chiropodist on duty. It is, however, also popular with the staff, as it provides an element of the unexpected, and a change in their usual routine. For the clerical staff it is also a popular innovation, as they now have a positive response to make when confronted by someone in pain. In addition, they are no longer seen as refusing access to treatment: if treatment is denied, it is by the chiropodist.

As said above, the application form has also been redesigned. In the combined form for professionals and self-referrals, the section relating to foot condition has been expanded, whilst the medical history/treatment section has been simplified. A scale of urgency has also been introduced, and it is planned to test the accuracy of referrers' opinions against those of chiropodists.

The waiting list is to be one of the first things to be put on the computerised appointment system. This will save much hunting through files for the relevant pieces of paper and will give details such as date of first application, date of assessment and the outcome of that appointment. The computer will also be able to give an immediate display of the length of the assessed list for any given clinic. In turn, this will allow the clerical staff to give enquirers a more accurate estimation of the position in relation to receiving treatment. This is all theoretically possible now, but very time consuming.

Thus, whilst the waiting list has not been abolished, there is now a much more equitable system and, for those most in need, almost instant access to a chiropodist.

The improvement in the previous administrative system will help reduce the size of the list and bring some relief to those who still must wait. But this study of the waiting list must be set in the broader context of all the other studies done on unmet need. When people talk about waiting lists, the first, most common and understandable comment is on their excessive length. But the footcare needs of people out in the community– the quiet ones who make no application for chiropody treatment – were also investigated. Among them substantial unmet need for footcare was found – need much, much greater than that represented by the waiting list. These people too need treatment; they too are in a sense waiting, silently and in their own homes. It is not necessarily those who apply who have the severest need. The formal waiting list is just the visible end of a very long queue for footcare. The longest portion waits in stoicism.

Part III

Current Provision: Insufficient and Inefficient

13 Mismatching problems and personnel

Discovery of unmet need on the scale found in this study has serious implications, for national health policy and for everyone involved in the provision of footcare. Put bluntly, the present strategy for dealing with foot problems will never succeed.

For several years it has been recognised, as noted in the first chapter, that existing footcare manpower is grossly inadequate to meet current demand. Government's response has been to increase the number of fully-trained chiropodists, establishing two new schools of chiropody. In itself, this is commendable. Britain certainly needs more chiropodists and governments have been willing to invest substantial funds in new training facilities at a time when most public expenditure was being restrained. But expansion of skilled manpower will not suffice to deal with the problem.

The previous calculations of manpower shortages showed that the National Health Service has less than half the chiropodists it needs. But even this dramatic shortfall was based on a restricted concept of need. The estimates were concerned basically with providing a service for elderly people, and assumed that only half the pension age population needed footcare. The present research suggests a much higher incidence of foot problems among elderly people and substantial unmet need for footcare among other vulnerable groups. And the needs of the majority of the population which is effectively excluded from NHS chiropody under the present rationing system of priority groups could not even be considered. There is no hope that increasing the number of professional chiropodists will ever cope with the full need for footcare in Britain.

How footcare is provided and who provides it must be considered afresh. Can the efficiency of foot health services be substantially raised? Can substantial new sources of manpower be raised? Can this be done without raising costs? These are the questions confronted in the second part of the study, an investigation of the current provision of footcare.

In the Footcare Spectrum (see page 17) a range of problems of the foot was set along a continuum of increasing seriousness, paralleled by a range of increasingly skilled people to deal with them – nurses, physiotherapists, chiropodists, doctors, surgeons. One aim of any treatment service is a cost-effective matching of problems and personnel. One important and recurrent form of inefficiency in health care provision is the use of high skill (and hence high cost) personnel to deal with simple problems that do not require their level of competence. This not only raises the cost of treatment, absorbing resources which could be used to expand the service elsewhere, but also means that patients with more complex problems have to wait for treatment because the appropriate, highly skilled personnel are engaged on other work. Thus, one general focus of the investigation into inefficiency in current footcare provision was on how patients are allocated and referred between the possible treaters, the appropriateness of the match between problems and personnel.

Matching more complex

Recent improvements in the recognised training of chiropodists have made the problems of matching more complex, but also created new opportunities for increased efficiency. Chiropodists are now qualified to administer local analgesics, do minor surgery and use advanced technology treatments like cryotherapy and ultra-sound. Thus, they are now able to treat a larger range of foot problems, including some that could previously only be dealt with by doctors. Yet they are still considerably less expensive to train and to employ than doctors. This creates the potential for savings through allocating foot patients to chiropodists rather than doctors. This possibility guided the research. The resources were not available to study all types of footcare provision, so attention was concentrated on the relationship between chiropodists and the three principal types of doctor involved in footcare, general practitioners, accident and emergency departments, and surgeons.

Shifting new patients to an already overburdened chiropody service, however cost-effective this might be in theory, would only create additional problems, unless there were a radical improvement in the efficiency of chiropodists. Because chiropodists are the specialists in footcare it was decided to make them the subject of a much more comprehensive efficiency investigation, covering the effectiveness as well as the organisation of treatment.

But the issue of mismatching problems to personnel arises within chiropody too. While the training has improved greatly, many practising chiropodists spend much of their time giving routine palliative treatments and even basic foot hygiene. Much of this treatment could be provided, in a more cost-effective way, by people with a very much briefer and less expensive training.

Possibility hardly exists

At present, the possibility of matching the less serious foot problems with appropriate personnel hardly exists. As mentioned earlier, there is intense controversy with the chiropody profession about the use of footcare assistants and voluntary agencies to provide basic services. While this debate continues, the expansion of these new sources of manpower has been effectively blocked. Thus, we are faced with an economic opportunity and a practical problem: the development of new roles in the sub-chiropodial section of the footcare spectrum.

Because this issue is central to dealing with unmet need, it was made the focus of special attention. In investigating chiropody services, the extent to which the existing workload could be delegated to sub-chiropodial roles was measured. Then, the practicalities of their development was considered.

In sum, the point has been reached when Britain's footcare strategy must be re-thought and then re-shaped. This involves both eliminating problems in the present ways of doing things and realising the potential of new approaches.

14 General practitioners:
under-detection and under-referral

Family doctors are the first port of call for most people with most of their health problems. Thus they become the key to footcare provision, both in terms of detecting need and in allocating problems to personnel.

The general practitioner's first task is to diagnose the problem the patient presents to him. But he may or may not then go on further to detect additional felt and potential needs, including needs for footcare.

Having recognised problems, the doctor may then choose to treat them himself or refer them on to others. This allocation decision is crucial for the efficiency of the footcare services. His choice among options for referral will depend, in part, on the nature of the problem, but also on his knowledge of, attitude towards, and relationships with, the other providers of footcare. He may make an appropriate, cost-effective referral. Alternatively, he may choose someone incapable of dealing with the problem or, more likely, someone more highly trained and more costly than necessary. In sum, there are two potential problems in general practitioners' approach to footcare: what they miss as well as what they do, questions of detection, then questions of referral.

Before beginning the research, there were reasons for believing that both types of problem exist. The pressure under which most general practitioners work, with an average consultation of only six minutes per patient, means that they have little enough time to deal with the problems which are presented to them, much less seek out others. Felt needs will likely remain unexpressed, potential needs remain undiscovered. These are the problems of omission.

Problems of commission

The problems of commission are somewhat more visible. The existing pattern of referrals from GPs to chiropodists is extremely restricted, mainly elderly and handicapped patients with a narrow range of simple foot problems – toenails, corns and callouses. General practitioners are thus making use of only a very small portion of chiropodists' skills. This is consistent with other research on doctors, which showed that they had only limited knowledge of chiropody and even more limited contact with chiropodists, and hence saw them as competent to treat only a limited set of conditions (Winkler and Paley, 1983). But then, what do general practitioners do with the non-priority group patients they encounter, and with the more serious foot problems? Do they, as with so much else, send them to hospital?

Ideally both sorts of problem should have been studied. But that would have required conducting interviews and foot examinations with a large sample of patients attending a representative range of general practices. Such a study was well beyond the resources available. So it was decided to concentrate on how family doctors deal with the foot problems presented to them, and consider only indirectly the extent to which they detect additional conditions.

The research consisted in tracing what happened to all patients with foot problems who attended a selected health centre during one week. An investigation specifically directed towards foot problems will inevitably sensitise doctors to look for them, however much they are asked to work normally. There is no way of eliminating this effect, so it was maximised. A particularly 'good' health centre was chosen for study, that is, one with a reputation for having caring doctors, with a record of collaboration with other health professionals, with excellent modern facilities including the headquarters of the chiropody service directly off the doctors' waiting room, and one where positive, co-operative relationships exist between the general practitioners and the chiropodists. It was a study of best practice. If there were problems and inefficiencies here, they would be much greater in normal conditions.

For every patient attending during the week, a special form was prepared. The age and sex of the patient was recorded at the top. These forms were then inserted into the patients' notes by the reception staff. At the consultation, the doctor then filled in the remaining three question section of the form. The first question was a simple yes/no to 'Did this patient present with, or did you diagnose, any condition of the feet?' If the answer was 'yes', the doctor then ticked the appropriate diagnosis from a list. Finally, he indicated what action he had taken, including a referral if any.

During the study week, 263 people attended to see a doctor. Of these, only 11 (4.2%) either consulted about, or had diagnosed, a problem of the feet. And despite the survey, which alerted doctors to the potential use of chiropodists, only two people were actually referred for chiropody. The pattern of treatment for all these patients was as follows:

Table 18: General practitioners' responses to foot problems

Referral back to hospital (as 'old' patients)	4
Referral to hospital as new patients	1
Referral to chiropody department	2
Treated by the general practitioner	3
Condition and action not recorded	1
TOTAL	11

Of the ten whose condition was recorded, six were clearly within the scope of a state registered chiropodist. These included the two patients referred, both of whom had callosities, two cases of fungal infections, one *verruca* (wart) and one patient who needed a new arch support.

Of the remaining four, one patient had an ulcer on the foot and was receiving hospital treatment. Another had a diabetic foot ulcer which could have benefitted from chiropody in conjunction with the diabetic clinic. The two remaining patients had swollen feet and the GP was observing progress rather than taking an active role. None of these four could have been treated by a chiropodist alone, although he could advise on swelling and treat the ulcer in co-ordination with others. If they had come to a chiropodist directly, the usual course of action would be for him to diagnose, treat locally and refer for further investigation.

Because the sample was so small, it had been intended to supplement these results with an anlysis of the GPs' past referrals. This proved impossible for two revealing reasons. First, urgent referrals had been dealt with and the forms put away in the patient's chiropody notes, so no comprehensive record existed of GPs' referrals. Second, the referral forms were designed in such a way that medical conditions were commonly given, whilst foot conditions were frequently omitted. The analysis was thus impossible. But the discovery of exactly how and why the existing referral forms were inadequate stimulated the design of a new form, which is now in use in the district.

Doctors refer to hospitals

From the very small sample thus available from the week's study, doctors appear to have a limited view of the scope of chiropodists, which leads them to make much less use of the chiropody service than is appropriate on both cost and therapeutic grounds. Their preferred option for foot problems is referral to hospital. This is doubly costly. The use of hospital resources to treat conditions within a chiropodist's scope needlessly increases costs to the NHS. It also costs the patient extra time and trouble. Instead of walking across the hall to chiropody, he or she has to make a special appointment for separate treatment in another institution. These patient costs are usually excluded from health service calculations because the NHS does not have to pay them. But they constitute a deterrent to use of the health service and hence are one important factor in creating the high levels of unmet need which were discovered.

The second most popular course of action for the doctor was to treat some conditions himself. In some cases, this is not only the most appropriate action, but also the quickest, But, for other conditions, chiropodists have access to equipment which is not available to the average family doctor. More generally, delegation of foot problems leaves doctors time to give to other patients for whom the chiropodist can do nothing. When the chiropodists are as convenient as they were in this health centre, this is an efficient way to use specialised skills, in terms of everyone's time, as well as money. There is an additional gain, however. When new patients are referred, chiropodists will, as a matter of routine practice, conduct a thorough examination of the foot, looking for all problems, not just those which the patient presented. It is a limited, but easy and inexpensive way of detecting and dealing with unmet need. That leads directly on to the next finding from the health centre study.

The low rate of referral is only one issue. A much greater problem is the low detection of foot problems among patients attending their GP. While inefficient referral is of concern to the NHS, for the patients it is the non-recognition of their foot problems which is of most concern.

The resources were not available to conduct the foot examinations which would have provided a quantified estimate of the extent to which doctors failed to detect foot problems. But it was demonstrated in the unmet need studies of both elderly people and children that an enormous number of foot problems will be found if a professionally trained person has the time to examine feet. Amongst elderly people, 88% had some problem, including 25% who were not receiving any form of treatment whatsoever. Among the schoolchildren, 91% needed advice or treatment for problems with feet or footwear. During the week in question, these two groups alone would have produced more problems than were recorded by the GPs. This, then, is *prima facie* evidence of a gross under-recognition of foot problems, illustrating the urgent necessity of further research on a much larger scale.

To acknowledge this under-recognition openly is not to find fault with general practitioners. The conditions in which most GPs practice, even in the selected modern health centre, mean that they do not have the time, and hence neither the inclination, to carry out the necessary foot examinations. Nor is there an easy way to incorporate such an examination into the investigation of other conditions, since it is rare for patients to remove their shoes and hose when consulting the doctor. But detecting unmet need for footcare remains a major task and examining patients who have already come into contact with the health service through their general practitioner is one of the easier and more logical ways to go about it.

Findings confirm suspicions

The findings of this small research project have lent confirmation to both the problems which it was suspected existed. There are two major issues at stake; how to increase the detection of foot problems and how to improve the level of referrals to chiropodists.

The answer to the first is, in theory, clear: screen patients attending GP surgeries. In practice, there are still several serious decisions to be made. Who would do the screening? The obvious candidates are doctors, district or clinical nurses, and chiropodists. All are at present more than fully occupied. Who would be screened? One could examine all patients. Or one could limit the number who have to be dealt with by concentrating on specific vulnerable groups, such as those starting school, those who become pregnant, or those reaching retiring age. This would ease the manpower problem at the cost of rationing screening for an already rationed service. Finally, there is the question of whether screening should be automatic or voluntary, a matter of social as well as health policy.

Behind all these decisions lie resource constraints, in terms of money, time and manpower. Under the current financial restraints, no new resources are likely to be available to provide an extra service. This is actually a blessing. No matter who provided it, on whatever restricted terms, a screening service for foot problems is likely to be successful, too successful; that is, it would discover more genuine need for footcare than the chiropody service as presently organised could cope with.

Until such time as the waiting list has been eliminated and the proportion of patients requiring routine treatment for life has been reduced, it would be premature to start such a programme. Screening is a policy for the future.

There is, however, something which could be done now: to start improving the knowledge which doctors have about the scope of practice of chiropodists and about the type of services they provide. This would lead to a modest increase in referrals, reducing the use of expensive hospital facilities for the NHS, reducing the inconvenience for patients, and making a small dent in the problem of unmet need. Given the low detection of foot problems by general practitioners, the chiropody service could probably cope with this limited increase in its work load.

In the longer term, improved communications between the two professions and reforms in the chiropody service described in Chapter 23 would lay the basis for gradually increasing co-operation, leading towards a comprehensive service when a screening programme becomes practicable.

15 Accident and emergency departments: opportunity overlooked

'Accident and emergency departments' (A & E departments) in Britain today are misnamed. To be sure they do treat the victims of genuine accidents, emergencies and casualties. But they are also one of the few hospital departments which people may attend without an appointment or referral. In parts of the country, particularly urban areas, many patients take their general, non-emergency health problems directly to the hospital, rather than going first to their family doctor. This pattern of use is reinforced because general practitioners themselves often refer patients to the A & E for diagnostic x-rays and minor surgical treatments that are beyond their own resources. The consequence is that many A & E departments have evolved into a surrogate, supplementary and expanded form of general practice.

This is an expensive way to provide the first contact or primary care part of a health service. And not only in terms of money. A & E departments are frequently overcrowded places, with long waiting times for patients and relentless work pressure on staff. The immediately relevant consequence of this pattern of use is that many relatively minor foot problems are presented to A & E departments. The questions are: how many? how do the doctors there deal with them? could chiropodists have dealt with them as well, at lower cost?

The research was conducted in the A & E department of the highly reputed teaching hospital in the district. In this hospital, the chiropody service is located immediately adjacent to 'casualty', in the same main entrance hall. Once again, the health service was being studied in optimum conditions for co-operation and cross-referral between those who provide footcare.

The broad design of the investigation was that every patient who presented at the registration desk with any problem of the foot or lower leg (below the knee) was followed through the department to observe the diagnostic procedures and treatment given. As far as possible, the researchers (who were all qualified chiropodists) did not interfere with the normal course of events. The recording schedules were designed to allow collection of the required information simply by watching the natural progression of the patient through the department.

Again, this research design was a compromise. Ideally, foot examinations on all patients coming to the department should have been conducted, as a measure both of unmet need in the general population and of the extent to which doctors were missing foot problems. But with some 200 patients a day passing through the casualty department, this was well beyond the resources available. However, the observational study did allow the authors to note whether doctors went beyond the presenting problem to look for other foot conditions.

All patients coming to the A & E department report first to a registration desk, whether it is their initial or a subsequent visit. For first visits, details of name, address, age and injury are recorded in a large register. By arrangement with the registration clerks, a coloured dot was stuck in the book for every leg or foot problem to ensure that no patients were missed. The casualty notes of all patients were similarly tagged so that information could be extracted from them later if necessary.

Ideally, the chiropodist-researchers met the patients at the registration desk, completing the first part of the schedule (concerning background information) as the registration clerk questioned them. It is at this point that any referral letters are handed in, allowing the researchers to identify why the patient attended. If this was not spontaneously made clear, the patient was asked why he decided to attend: was it his own idea? was he advised to attend? if so, by whom?

The patient is then seen by a doctor who may make a diagnosis immediately or send the patient for an x-ray, making a final diagnosis when the x-rays are returned. Treatment is then given as appropriate, often by nurses. The patient may be discharged, told to visit his general practitioner, or scheduled for a return appointment at casualty. He may also be admitted to hospital or sent to another department.

The researchers recorded not only the final diagnosis, but also the procedures taken to reach it (palpation, testing of movements, x-rays, etc,), to see how many were within the scope of practice of chiropodists. Note was taken of the treatment given (including advice) and by whom. The chiropodist-researchers also recorded the diagnosis and treatment-or-referral which they would have given if the patient had presented directly to them. In this district it is possible for patients to do this without referral from another source, so diagnoses could be compared.

These facts gave a detailed picture of the types of foot conditions dealt with by the A & E department and so it was possible to estimate how many of them could have been treated by a chiropodist, if they had been referred. This is a rough indicator of the mismatch of problems to personnel.

A total of 1,154 people attended during the week of the survey. Of them, 60 presented with problems of the leg or foot, 5.2% of the cases. Most were relatively minor conditions, yet 88% of these patients were self-referrals, people who chose to come directly to the hospital rather than going to their GP or to a chiropodist.

With certain important qualifications, most of the 60 could have been dealt with adequately by a state registered chiropodist. Certainly, all the problems presented were ones which chiropodists regularly encounter in their surgeries already. In fact, only one case was referred for chiropody. This represents an enormous under-use of a specialist resource and hence a potential for savings by the NHS.

The qualifications are that, if chiropodists are to be more closely integrated with casualty departments, they would need regularised access to:

medical back-up for some diagnoses and for prescribing restricted drugs;

support services in the form of x-ray facilities, pathology laboratories, and nursing assistance.

How and why chiropodists would need to use these services will become clear from the detailed analysis of the foot problems presented at the A & E department.

Foot problems presented

Soft tissue injuries

Soft tissue injuries include bruises, cuts, strains and sprains. There were 43 such cases during the week, 72% of the total leg and foot injuries. Most of these could have been both diagnosed and treated by a chiropodist. But most chiropodists do not have direct access to the technical aids used to confirm or exclude diagnoses. The majority (35 cases) were injuries of the ankle and tarsus, caused by falling or twisting movements. In all but the simplest cases, the A & E doctors requested x-rays to rule out the possibility of a fracture diagnosis. In no case was a fracture confirmed; that is to say, in no case was the clinical diagnosis proved wrong. It would appear that x-rays are requested for medico-legal reasons, to confirm rather than provide the diagnosis. Of all the soft tissue injuries, only four (three puncture wounds and one deep vein thrombosis) were beyond the scope of a chiropodist for treatment.

Bony injuries and conditions

Nine patients presented problems involving bone during the week. Three had bone conditions which definitely required medical advice, supervision and treatment. The others suspected they had broken a bone and, quite rightly, expected to see a doctor and have their condition diagnosed by x-ray. One stress fracture had already healed. The other five fractures were of a minor nature, none requiring plaster casts and all were treated simply by elastic strapping.

Infections

Four cases of infection were seen during the week, two bacterial, one fungal, one viral. All were of the sort frequently encountered in chiropody practice, all within the scope of a state registered chiropodist. There was a relevant complication in the case of the patient with the fungal infection, who was returning for a second visit. On his first attendance an apparently septic blister was opened and the contents sent to the pathology laboratory for testing. Here again, not all chiropodists have direct access to the facilities of such a laboratory. The case of the virus infection, plantar warts, was revealing in a different way. This was the one patient referred to the chiropody department. In fact, she was already receiving private chiropody and had only come to the A & E department because her chiropodist was ill.

Nail cases

All the four cases of problems with toenails were well within the scope of chiropodists. None were referred to the chiropody department.

In contrast to the making of diagnoses, the actual treatments were mostly carried out by nurses. Only four cases (tetanus toxin injections) were beyond the scope of chiropodists. All the remaining treatments were dressings or strappings, with advice on rest.

To summarise, chiropodists could have relieved the A & E department of most of its foot patients, some 5% of its workload. Why then did the department not make more use of the chiropodists? There are many possible explanations. One may be ignorance of the scope of practice of chiropodists. Doctors are often not aware of the recent improvements in chiropody training. If this was the reason, then it is yet another justification for an extensive programme to educate doctors about the current competence of chiropodists.

Conversely, non-referral may have been a conscious decision by the casualty doctors because they prefer to intervene themselves or delegate to the nurses who work with them. In the overcrowded conditions of the A & E department, one would have thought doctors would welcome every extra resource they could get. In any case, they need to be made aware of the extra costs they incur by not involving the chiropody service. Doctors do not receive much training in the economics of their work, so information on the comparative costs of A & E and chiropody services could be beneficial for all sides. Hospital administrators, who are concerned about cost control, could provide it.

The fact that the research was carried out in a teaching hospital may have influenced decisions. Some medical school teachers consciously acquiesce in the misuse of A & E departments as surrogate general practices, on the grounds that students are thus brought to deal with a broader range of medical problems. Referral to others is not encouraged, so that students may receive a more comprehensive training. It is an expensive lesson, a training in the inefficient use of resources.

The training function exacerbates another characteristic of A & E departments, a high turnover of medical staff. In this particular hospital there is a frequent changeover of both students and doctors. Any personal understandings and co-operative arrangements developed between individual chiropodists and doctors will thereby be regularly disrupted and short-lived. The implication of this is that the role of the chiropodist in the A & E department must be formally institutionalised and newcomers systematically inducted into the working arrangements.

Most perverse but most probable is non-referral through oversight. While knowing that a chiropodist could help, the A & E doctors may simply have overlooked the availability of chiropody, even though it is literally right next door. The A & E department is almost a self-contained world. It has it own reception desk, its own x-ray facilities, its own minor surgery room. Most of the services it needs are located within the department itself, administered by the department's own staff. The chiropody service is located just the other side of the boundary. The physical distance may be short, but the social distance is enormous.

The pre-requisite for efficient co-operation between the two services, therefore, is that a chiropodist must be physically located within the A & E department. The individuals may rotate, but a chiropody service should become an integral part of the department's resources and chiropodists be seen as members of the A & E team.

Organisation of integration

The next step is to give the chiropodist access to the support services needed to do the job thoroughly. This means, specifically, the right to order x-rays, the right to order pathology laboratory tests, and the right to call on nursing assistance in treatment. These rights would be exercised in consultation with A & E doctors, and according to current agreements between the Society of Chiropodists and the relevant medical/surgical organisations. In fact, this is already common practice under informal arrangements between some individual chiropodists and doctors, but they would need to be formalised in order to avoid recurrent delays. The actual organisation of integration, which functions the chiropodist would assume, may vary and develop over time. Two broad options seem feasible.

1. Doctors diagnose, chiropodists treat

After diagnosing a foot problem in the normal way, A & E staff could pass the patient on to a chiropodist for immediate treatment, in much the same way as they already refer patients with speech problems to a speech therapist.

While chiropodists are trained in a much more restricted field than doctors, they have both expertise and much experience in dealing with the foot problems that come within their scope of practice. Through a referral-for-treatment system, the chiropodist could contribute his skills to the A & E department, while having its back-up. This would cut waiting time for patients and ease the work load for casualty doctors.

And here again, the chiropodist would conduct a thorough foot examination, looking for additional problems. This would be a valuable supplement to the existing A & E service. In no instance during the research did the casualty doctors appear to look for any other foot problems than those presented to them. Certainly in no case did they diagnose or treat any other foot condition.

In one sense this is understandable and proper. After all, it was an emergency service, designed to deal with immediate problems not to offer general medical treatment, that was being studied. And the pressure under which A & E departments work means there is scant time to go beyond the immediate. On the other hand, one of the difficulties in discovering unmet need for footcare, is that the feet are so seldom exposed to people who can recognise pathological conditions. When patients spontaneously contact the health service with a foot problem this is an opportunity for a more general inspection not to be missed. We cannot realistically expect A & E doctors to undertake such additional work. But if all foot patients were referred to chiropodists for treatment, it would become a matter of normal routine.

Such a referral system is a practical possibility, indeed it already exists. Shortly after the fieldwork for this research was completed, the district chiropody headquarters moved into new premises in a hospital, next door to the casualty department. Contacts were immediately established with the orthopaedic consultant in charge of the department and a system of referral-for-treatment was established, including surgical interventions like toenail removals (which are discussed in detail on pages 100 to 101).

Extending such co-operative arrangements to a normal hospital would be more complex. But chiropodists already work in hospitals on a regular basis, both in wards and in clinics. Compared to the many other problems which beset the footcare services, providing treatment facilities in support of A & E departments would be relatively easy to organise.

2. *Chiropodists as first contact*

A more extensive form of co-operation would involve all patients who present at an A & E department with foot problems being sent directly to chiropodists for preliminary diagnosis. In fact, chiropodists are doing this job already – in their own surgeries. Under present arrangements, chiropodists are trained to recognise all the problems of the foot. They are trained, as well, to recognise which are within their competence to treat alone, and which they must refer on for specialist medical attention. And, as the results from one of the other studies will show (see page 158), they tend to take a conservative view of their scope of practice, restricting rather than enlarging their interventions.

Patients can and do refer themselves for chiropody treatment without a doctor's letter, just as they do to casualty. It is for this reason that chiropodists already see the full range of problems which were presented at the A & E department – and more besides. They diagnose them, treat and/or refer them as part of their regular work, and they diagnose accurately. In all of the 60 cases studied here, the chiropodist-researchers reached the same diagnosis as the casualty doctors.

Doing this diagnostic task as part of an A & E department would only be an extension of work chiropodists do already, but it would make a novel and substantial contribution to easing the workload of A & E departments. They would need the support of hospital services and medical back-up for some final diagnoses and treatments. But there is more than merely potential for a better service here. It already exists in some areas in a fragmentary and unstructured way. Co-operation and cross-referral between chiropodists and casualty departments just needs to be openly recognised, positively organised and made regular practice.

16 Surgeons: a waste of skill

Surgeons are the most costly group of professional staff within the NHS. They are expensive, not only because of the salaries they command, but also because of the length of their training, and most importantly, because of the facilities and support they require to do much of their work – operating theatres stocked with sophisticated equipment, anaesthetists, nurses and assistants during operations, and recuperative beds in hospital for their patients afterwards.

It is therefore economically sensible (apart from any other considerations) that they should spend their working lives performing operations which require a fully-fledged surgeon. However, minor operations are still carried out by surgeons which could be done by less extensively trained personnel in less expensive surroundings. In the area of foot problems, surgeons are still engaged in, for example, the removal of *verrucae* and toenails.

Most of the operations carried out by surgeons on the legs and feet are clearly beyond the scope of a state registered chiropodist. Over the past decade, however, more radical procedures have been increasingly introduced into the training of chiropodists, including nail avulsions (removals). Nonetheless, the development of chiropodial surgery is still at an early stage in Britain. In the United States, chiropodists undergo an extra three years training and are known, more logically, as 'podiatrists', they can already perform a broad range of operations, including arthodesis, digital (toe) straightening, and *hallux valgus* operations. Several groups are pressing for a similar extension to chiropodists' skills here.

But surgeons in Britain are divided over the transfer of even straightforward toenail operations to chiropodists. Some object in the mistaken belief that chiropodists are incapable of such work, while others seek to preserve a source of private practice. In contrast, another group sees referral of these operations simply as an efficient division of labour and affirms the judgement of an eminent surgeon who wrote in *The Lancet*, '. . . in the context of present-day standards of nail surgery, many patients might be better off having germinal matrix phenolised by a skilled chiropodist'. (Fowler, 1975).

The fact is that, at present, the removal of ingrown or deformed toenails, either totally or a side section(s), is part of a state registered chiropodist's scope of practice. So is the destruction of the matrix (growing area of the toenail) by chemical or electrical cautery. This is done under a local anaesthetic injected into the offending toe. In contrast with most surgical techniques, it does not even involve cutting through the skin. The operation takes less than 20 minutes and is done as an outpatient procedure. The patient has to come back to the clinic regularly for dressings, but usually returns to work or school the day after the procedure.

Obviously, there are patients for whom such a procedure would be unwise – those with peripheral neuropathy (loss of feeling) or with poor circulation in the foot and toes. For some patients, their medical history or treatment would make local anaesthesia or outpatient treatment inappropriate. But part of chiropodists' training is in recognising the complications to apparently simple foot problems caused by other medical conditions. When they encounter a combination of conditions which possibly puts a problem beyond a chiropodist's scope of practice, they seek medical advice before either proceeding or referring on to surgeons.

However, for the average person, having an ingrown toenail removed under local anaesthesia by a chiropodist is no more traumatic than a trip to the dentist, which also involves local anaesthesia. Indeed, for many, it is fa less traumatic, since they can talk during the treatment, and many even choose to watch while reclining in the chiropodial chair.

Whoever performs the surgery, an additional problem may develop. Some toenail removals are completely successful. But in other cases the nail regrows in a thickened or distorted state, gradually becoming extremely uncomfortable. The problem may arise less frequently following removals by chiropodists, firstly because they use a different technique, and then because they provide their own aftercare, monitor the regrowth of the nail, and can intervene again at an early stage if necessary. Surgeons seldom see their failures, however, in part because they rarely provide their own aftercare, in part because patients often go to chiropodists for relief as the new nail becomes painful. Almost all chiropodists have such patients among their caseload. The problem could be dealt with by a further removal with destruction of the root matrix to prevent regrowth. But, not surprisingly, many of these patients are reluctant to consent to another operation, having already experienced a failure, especially if it involves a second trip back into hospital. In consequence they require regular palliative chiropody for the rest of their lives.

The point is that in this area of minor surgery, two types of footcare professionals are trained to deal with the same problems. The chiropodist has a much more restricted range of operating skills than the surgeon, but is competent within those limits. In some ways, because of the aftercare he provides, the total service provided by the chiropodist may be superior in a technical sense. In terms of direct costs to the NHS, it is vastly cheaper.

It costs the patient less too. For a hospital operation, the patient pays in time, and thrice over. Most surgeons have waiting lists and in their repertoire of skills toenail removals count as 'minor' operations. The result is that patients usually have to wait first for a consultation, then for the operation, and finally may have to spend time in hospital for recuperation. Commonly, this waiting time runs into months, sometimes even years. For much of this time the patient may be in pain, with restricted mobility which affects the way he conducts his life and work.

Chiropodists have waiting lists too. But they usually give patients with ingrown toenails priority. Much of a chiropodist's time is spent in repetitive, palliative work, but with this condition there is an opportunity for permanent cure and discharge. The motivation and job satisfaction in doing such work is high. The result is that the process of toenail removal by chiropodists, from first consultation to operation, usually takes only a matter of days.

It is difficult to quantify the cost of patients' waiting time, but we do have good measures of both the incidence and cost of ingrown toenail operations carried out by surgeons and chiropodists. The chiropody service maintains its own statistics on this procedure. The Hospital Activities Analysis (HAA), compiled for the Regional Health Authority, contains annual figures for such operations within the research district. The HAA statistics show: the operation carried out, the age and sex of the patient, the length of the admission, and the diagnoses, both primary diagnosis and any other (for example, *diabetes mellitus*). These figures are not complete, since they exclude procedures performed in A & E departments. But they cover all patients admitted to a day ward or overnight, and thus provide a basis for the most important comparison.

During the last year for which information was available (1978), 32 total or partial nail avulsions (removals) were undertaken by the district's chiropodists, while 73 hospital operations on toenails were carried out by surgeons. For seven of the hospital cases, a multiple diagnosis was recorded, including heart disease, diabetes and other medical problems requiring systemic medical treatment. Without tracing each individual it is not possible to say whether a chiropodist could have treated them or not. To minimise uncertainty and bias, we will assume all these patients genuinely required hospitalisation. This leaves 66 patients, without medical complications, who were nonetheless treated in hospital.

Roughly speaking, then, surgeons performed twice the number of straightforward in-grown toenail operations as chiropodists. This is a crude measure of the extent to which an operation, for which chiropodists are now trained, is still being carried out by surgeons. And this is some ten years since chiropodists have been accredited to conduct the procedure.

Behind these simple figures lies a substantial waste of training. Chiropodists are now trained in nail removal techniques but are precluded from doing this work because surgeons still pre-empt two thirds of the cases. And while surgeons are removing toenails, they are not performing the more sophisticated operations for which they alone are trained. Meanwhile the patients needing those operations wait. The loss is substantial. Those 66 toenail removals in hospital represent approximately 2 to 3 weeks of a surgeon's operating time.

Costs of alternative procedures

The greatest potential saving, however, becomes apparent on comparing the costs of the alternative procedures. The cost of toenail operations may be divided into three elements: operator costs, support costs and bed costs.

Operator costs

It is more expensive in salary terms for toenail operations to be carried out by surgeons than by chiropodists, but this is the least important of the cost elements. The procedure is normally done by a relatively senior chiropodist, but in hospital it will usually involve a registrar rather than a consultant. Assuming both are at the mid point of their careers, and leaving out complications like London Weighting and 'on-costs', the surgical registrar is paid £4.28 per hour and the Senior I chiropodist £3.60 per hour.

Both will have assistance. For the chiropodist it will usually be his junior, paid at £3.06 per hour. Even in the simplest hospital procedure, using local anaesthetic, the registrar would have the help of a staff nurse, at £2.61 per hour. While the operation itself may last only 20 minutes, if we include time for preparation, cleaning up and writing up notes, then the whole process may absorb roughly an hour. The operator costs in both cases are thus a little under £7.00.

Support costs

It is when surgeons opt for a general anaesthetic that costs are vastly increased. First, there would be the use of a operating theatre. Then there would be the cost of an anaesthetist, a theatre nurse, and other theatre staff involved in preparation and clearing away, plus porters. Without further detailed information on the 66 hospital operations, it is impossible to put an exact figure on these support costs. But theatre time for straightforward operations is costed at £45 per hour excluding staff. Thus, estimating conservatively, we may allow £60 per procedure for support costs, across the whole range of procedures used in hospital. The chiropodist's procedure is carried out in a specially reserved 'clean' room or a minor operations theatre, so that similar support costs do not occur.

Bed costs

Chiropodists do not admit patients for toenail procedures and thus incur no bed costs. The 66 patients dealt with by surgeons, however, spent varying amounts of time in hospital, from day ward admission which involves no overnight stay, to 12 days. There were 31 day ward cases. The other 35 patients spent 102 days in hospital, roughly three days each. The detailed distribution is shown in Table 19.

Table 19: Length of admissions for nail operations (1978)

(Figures denote number of people)

Age of patient	Day Ward	1	2	3	4	5	6	7	8	9	10	11	12	13	14	15 days
100																
90																
80		1														
70		3	1	1			2									
60		1			2	2										
50		2	2				1				1					
40		6	1													
30		3	2	1												
20		7	2	3	1	1										
10		8	6	3	1	1			1							

None of these patients were recorded as having a multiple diagnosis, so there is no known reason for admittance other than for the nail operation.

The cost of maintaining a patient in hospital is currently reckoned at £287 per week, or £41 per day. Thus, the 35 patients who were admitted overnight accounted for £4,182 bed costs (102 days x £41 per day). The cost of a day ward admission was estimated at half the cost of an overnight stay, ie. at £20 per day, The 31 patients admitted in this way absorbed £620 in bed costs. Together, all 66 hospital patients accounted for £4,802 in bed costs, or just under £73 apiece.

The following is a rough comparative costing of the alternative procedures:

	Surgeon £	Chiropodist £
Operator costs	7	7
Support costs	60	—
Bed costs	73	—
TOTAL COST	£140.00	£7.00

Thus the potential saving per procedure is £133. For all the 66 cases without medical complications, the total saving could thus have been at least £8,778. This is for one health district. There are 201 health districts in England and Wales. If a similar pattern existed throughout the country, then the potential saving on this one operation alone, in one year, is £1.76 million. Generalising from one health district to the nation involves a large measure of approximation, but clearly we are dealing here with a large misuse of resources and hence large potential savings.

While for such a 'minor' operation, this figure seems impressively large, it is useful to recall here what a limited calculation has just been made. There are no figures for operations done in hospitals at A & E departments, and no estimate of wasted training costs has been included, and no attempt has been made to assess the cost of patients' waiting time and other losses, neither those waiting for in-grown toenail operations, nor those waiting for the more serious operation which surgeons could have been doing. These are all real costs; no numbers can be put to them. They are also real potential savings.

Of all the inefficiencies in current footcare provision, this is apparently the simplest to deal with. The aim of policy should be to match problem to personnel, that is, to re-allocate all straight-forward in-grown toenail operations without medical complications away from surgeons to chiropodists. In practice, we are concerned here with the redefinition of professional roles and boundaries – always a complicated business. But the process can be carried out in stages.

Redefining professional roles

Part of the problem is simply a lack of information. Informal conversations with surgeons have revealed that many just did not know chiropodists were competent to perform ingrown toenail operations, and hence never even considered referring such patients to them. It is impossible for the authors to estimate how many surgeons are ill-informed in this way, but from conversations among chiropodists, they have reason to believe the number is large. For them, a concentrated information campaign is appropriate

Other surgeons know about chiropodists' training, but are sceptical about their competence to actually carry out the procedure. They need reassurance, and here the Royal College of Surgeons has a role to play. No amount of protesting from chiropodists will be as convincing to a surgeon as information provided by his own college. The Royal College approves examiners for the surgical examination taken at the end of the recognised training. It must make sure that its own members are convinced of chiropodists' competence in this area.

Regional health authorities and the Department of Health and Social Security could help as well, by informing hospital surgeons of the needless expense of their current procedures. Comparative data, such as that provided here, will convince the cost conscious. Others may need more active encouragement to transfer patients to chiropodists.

But for a long time yet, patients with ingrown toenails will find their way to hospital surgeons, if only because, as the present research has indicated in a small way, family doctors will send them there. Ensuring that such patients are then referred to chiropodists for treatment will depend, ultimately, on developing co-operative, trusting relationships between surgeons and chiropodists at the local level. Here chiropodists must assume the initiative. They have a lot to offer surgeons, in relieving work pressure, reducing waiting lists, and taking off their hands some 'minor' operations. If they then carry through the work competently, trust will grow, and out of trust, a regular pattern of referrals.

All this will take time. But chiropodists have been able to perform this operation for a decade now. It is time they were given the job to do.

17 Chiropody: the potential for change

The problem with the chiropody service is getting your foot in the door. At least, that is how the problem appears from the perspective of the patients. For all practical purposes, the only group with access to chiropody treatment on an individual basis is the elderly. Even for them there is a waiting list, which is so long and moves so slowly that many never even bother to join the queue.

The problem is just as frustrating to the providers as it is to the patients. There is a gross excess of demand for footcare over supply. The service wants to expand in order to deal with this unmet need. But it finds itself locked in to a pattern of giving so many repeated, palliative treatments to its existing patients, that it is unable to take on many new ones.

The imbalance between need and provision sets up a vicious circle. Because the NHS has only a small fraction of the chiropodists it needs, it must ration the footcare it provides to a few 'priority groups'. Many patients are thus driven to seek chiropody in the private sector. Chiropodists, those without formal state registration as much as those with it, can thus make a good living providing footcare privately. This makes it more difficult for the NHS to recruit and retain staff, forcing a further constriction of the service, creating waiting lists.

In theory, there are three possible strategies for breaking out of such a cycle of imbalanced supply and demand: reduce demand, increase supply, or raise the efficiency of providing the service. In chiropody, all are difficult.

With the elderly population increasing, there will actually be many more members of the 'priority group' in the near future who will require footcare services. As they already receive most of the available chiropody, there can be no compensatory drop in demand from any other sector of the population. Therefore, demand is likely to rise rather than fall.

The limiting factor on increasing the supply of chiropody is the shortage of manpower. In one recent survey, over half the district health authorities advertising for chiropodists did not receive a single applicant. As noted in Chapter 1, the private sector absorbs roughly half those with the state recognised qualification, and the recent small expansion of the chiropody schools (about 30 extra graduates a year in total) is likely to be offset by a surge in retirements over the next few years.

Increased efficiency

In the medium term ahead, therefore, the only realistic option is to increase efficiency. The DHSS gathers no statistics on the extent to which the chiropody services cure and discharge their patients. Analysis of the needs of elderly people and the waiting list (see Chapters 11 and 12) has indicated that if one waits until people reach pension age before dealing with their foot problems the most common reason for vacancies is not discharge but death.

The difficulty of curing their patients makes chiropodists despair and many gradually fall into a ritual of providing routine maintenance treatments. Turnover is low, few new patients are taken on, the service coagulates.

The structural problems faced by the chiropody services make expansion genuinely difficult. These difficulties produce in many of the professionals involved an understandable spirit of resignation. When the queue is endless, productivity seems pointless. In such an atmosphere, not only is there no incentive to remove blockages, but inefficient practices gradually become the tolerated norm. From experience of the service, the authors suspected three important forms of inefficiency had developed:

1. too little attempt to cure or improve conditions, leading to an excessive provision of routine maintenance treatments;

2. provision of these palliative treatments more frequently than necessary; and

3. the use of chiropodists to perform sub-chiropodial tasks.

All were found in abundance. But in reading the documentation of problems below, it should be constantly borne in mind that this research was conducted in a district which, by reputation and many other objective indicators, contains one of the best chiropody departments in the country. These then are the inefficiencies of the relatively efficient.

Inefficiencies of the relatively efficient

In broad outline, the research into these problems relied on making chiropodists re-consider their patients. Existing records were removed and analysed, and a profile of the care each patient had received over the preceding year was extracted. Then a new interview-examination schedule was substituted. Deprived of patient records, the chiropodists were forced to re-examine the person, make a fresh diagnosis and a new treatment decision. The schedules were then analysed and the old pattern compared with the new. The difference was simultaneously a measure of past routine and potential improvement.

In detail, this study was more complex than any of the others undertaken, including several sub-measures. First, the authors wanted a representative sample not only of patients, but also of the chiropodists who treated them and the clinics in which they were seen. It was decided that a complete census of all patients dealt with by the district chiropody service during one calendar week should be undertaken. Because of the repetitious nature of the work, there is little seasonality in chiropody, so the patients in any one week are a representative selection of the total caseload. A weekly study also covered all clinics and included both full and part-time chiropodists in exact proportion to the hours they normally work. A week was chosen in which no-one was on holiday. Fortunately it was also one in which no staff were absent through sickness. In total, 540 patients took part in the research during the week.

The clerical staff sent out appointments for the 'research week' in the usual way, no different from any other week. However, they extracted all the relevant patient records from the files. These were checked for any information which, if not disclosed to the chiropodists giving treatment, might prove dangerous to the patient or the staff. For example, a hepatitis carrier had an appointment during the week. All such data were transferred to the new, substitute schedules.

All chiropodists were then given a six-page interview-examination schedule for each of their patients that week, similar to those used in the elderly people and waiting list studies. In covering medical history and treatment, social factors, footwear and attitudes to footwear, it requested much more information than is normally recorded on a treatment card at a routine appointment. The chiropodists also noted the treatment they gave the patient and the date of the next appointment scheduled. Finally, here too, they recommended the treatment plan they considered most suitable for the patient, selecting from the list shown earlier and assuming all were possible.

One of the ritual forms of inefficiency in chiropody is known as the 'copy-on effect'. Because so much of their work is routine, it has long been suspected that chiropodists simply go on repeating the established pattern of care without actively considering if this is the optimum. They work from chiropodial diagnoses recorded long before, simply copy the last treatment recorded for each patient, and schedule the next appointment with the same interval (return period) as the last. This not only requires less thought and effort, it also avoids contention. Patients who have been receiving the same treatment for years often misunderstand and resist attempts to alter the pattern, especially if it involves any change in their footwear. This resistance actually increases if the chiropodist wants to attempt cure and discharge. Because of the waiting list, patients believe that if the condition recurs, they may have to wait a long time, perhaps a year or more, before they can get back into the service. They develop a justifiable fear of being discharged. Some chiropodists in turn, unconsciously develop a calculating attitude. If patients are discharged, their places are immediately taken by others who may have been waiting for a year and whose feet are in a terrible condition. There is a definite economy of effort in palliating the devil you know. The result is a tacit collusion between chiropodist and patient in repeating the familiar old treatments.

'Copying-on' impossible

By removing past records and forcing a fresh investigation, diagnosis and treatment, simple 'copying-on' was made impossible But to measure whether this produced any change, a base line had to be established to determine what the previous pattern of treatment had been. Therefore, each patient's records were analysed for:

- date of first treatment ever recorded;
- foot condition diagnosed;

- number of treatments in past 12 months;
- return periods between these treatments;
- pattern of past treatments (divided into the categories of Table 11).

The analysis of past records also made it possible for the pattern of care existing in the district's service before the research began to be documented. It confirmed in numbers the almost exclusive reliance on routine maintenance treatments. (Table 20).

Table 20: Distribution of patients by treatment plans obtained from existing records

1.	Advice appointment only	0.4	0.4	minimal treatment
2.	One treatment, then annual check up	0.0		
3.	One treatment, then discharge	0.0	0.4	curative treatment
4.	Intensive treatment, then discharge	0.4		
5.	Intensive treatment, then SOS only	0.7	0.7	occasional treatment
6.	Intensive treatment, then return intervals of 20 weeks or more	0.0		
7.	One treatment, then foot-care assistant	0.0	0.0	footcare assistance
8.	Intensive treatment, then footcare assistant	0.0		
9.	Intensive treatment, then routine maintenance	5.0	91.2	chiropody for life
10.	Routine maintenance	86.2		
11.	No decision recorded	7.2		

Here 91.2% of the patients are being given care which implies treatment for life. To be sure, up to the time of the research, the

district had never employed a footcare assistant, so this option was not available to the chiropodists. On the other had, the 7.2% of patients for whom the records were incomplete or illegible were very probably also routine maintenance cases. To put the point another way, only 1.5% of patients were definitely receiving any form of treatment other than routine maintenance.

While such a heavy use of maintenance treatments exceeded even the authors' suspicions, it does not, in and of itself, indicate inappropriate treatment. It might have been that the patients' feet had deteriorated, through childhood damage and years of neglect, to such an extent that no curative treatment was possible and palliation was the only answer. Therefore, it was decided that the extent to which routine maintenance was the appropriate treatment should be tested. To do this, the patients' foot conditions were categorised and compared with the treatment patterns. It was found that the conditions could be grouped into nine categories, as in Table 21.

Table 21: Types of foot condition

Nails only	ie	nails of normal thickness requiring cutting and filing only.
Acute	ie	acute inflammation, ulcers, infections.
Chronic serious	ie	ulcers slow to heal, sinuses, any long-standing condition liable to infection.
Chronic palliative	ie	conditions of long term nature, eg. callouses and corns, receiving the same treatment routinely.
Mixed	ie	variations between other categories too frequent to easily classify.
Nails plus 1 lesion	ie	nail cutting required plus use of scalpel but no padding applied.
Nails only but require drill	ie	thickened or distorted nails which require reduction in length and thickness.
Chiropody but progressive improvement	ie	corns, callouses etc, which through treatment show and continue to show improvement.
Nail avulsions	ie	patients who have had total or partial removal of nail(s) under local analgesia.

Of these conditions, the two chronic categories will probably always need long-term routine maintenance. But for all the other conditions, routine maintenance is probably the wrong answer. For example, those with nail problems only should, unless their medical history prevents it, be transferred to footcare. For those with only one lesion, a concerted attack on the cause of the problem might considerably reduce their long-term need for chiropody. For these other categories of conditions, then, some other treatment is, in principle, possible.

From the past records, the foot conditions for that 91.2% of the existing patients definitely receiving routine maintenance were analysed.

Table 22: Foot conditions of patients receiving routine maintenance

Category of Condition	No. of patients
Nails only	44
Acute	1
Chronic serious	22
Chronic palliative	267
Nails and 1 lesion	104
Nails requiring thinning	9
Chiropody with progressive improvement	6
Nail avulsions	0
Mixed	13
TOTAL	466

Some 62% of patients are in the two chronic categories. There is thus a substantial genuine need for routine maintenance treatment. But there are also 38% for whom there is probably a better answer. This is a rough, *prima facie* indicator of the overuse of routine maintenance.

Not only was it discovered that the service was giving inappropriate treatments, but it was giving them too frequently. This became clear from comparing the return periods (intervals between appointments) given to patients over the preceding year and the return periods recommended for these same patients during the research week.

Effect of excessively frequent treatments

It is not immediately obvious, even to chiropodists themselves, what a dramatic reduction in the total capacity of the service is produced by excessively frequent treatments. Table 23 shows the consequences. Under the current manpower norms, a full-time chiropodist gives approximately 3,600 treatments a year. If he sees each patient once a year, he will thus treat 3,600 different people. If he sees each patient twice a year, that is, with a return period of 26 weeks, he will see 1,800 different people. The table shows the total number of different people who would be seen in a year if given various intervals between appointments.

Table 23: Caseload variation caused by differing return periods

Treatments per year	Interval between Appointments (in weeks)	Total patients seen
	52	3,600
	26	1,800
	16	1,107
3600	12	830
	10	691
	8	553
	6	415
	4	277

Thus, if every patient is seen even two weeks earlier than necessary, for example waiting only six weeks rather than eight, then 138 fewer patients (553 to 415) will be seen by that chiropodist. At the time of the research, the district was employing the equivalent of 14.4 full-time clinical chiropodists. A fortnight's reduction in the return periods they scheduled for their patients would mean that 1,987 people would remain unseen. This is more than twice the length of the waiting list.

There is, then, good reason to check the frequency with which patients are treated. This is not to advocate stretching the interval between appointments beyond what is clinically appropriate. There can be benefits from short term periods. If patients are seen at short intervals, there may be less treatment to be given, since lesions will not have had time to deteriorate. Short return periods, scheduled as part of an intensive treatment programme, may lead to the cure and discharge of the patient, or at least to less frequent maintenance visits. Nonetheless, the apprehension remained that chiropodists were simply copying the previous return period, rather than making a fresh assessment of the condition of the feet at each visit. Again, they are encouraged in this by patients. Frequent visits do not just minimise the risk of discomfort. The caring attitude and physical contact involved in chiropody treatments are valuable to many old people. Again, an unarticulated agreement develops between chiropodists and patients for short return periods.

Average return period

Of the total sample, it was possible to calculate from existing records the average return period over the preceding year for 519 patients. However, in 127 cases, there had been a change in the patient's condition between the research week and the preceding treatment. These were left out of the analysis because an alteration in the return period might have been appropriate in these cases. In order to test whether, as a result of the fresh reconsideration of patients forced on the chiropodists during the research week, the frequency of visits changed even though the patients' condition had not, only the 392 patients with stable conditions were included in the analysis.

In only 27% of the cases was the recommended new return period the same as that prevailing over the previous year. These people were thus being seen at the right intervals in the chiropodists' opinion. The remaining 73% is a rough indicator of the copying-on effect.

For 22% of the cases, the recommendation was actually shorter than the past average. This would result in more treatment. But most of these shorter return periods were probably recommended as part of intensive treatment programmes designed to reduce visits over the long-term. The chiropodists were not just proposing the same old treatments more often.

In exactly 50% of the cases, the recommendation was for a longer interval between appointments than before. On balance, therefore, there would be a substantial reduction in the total number of treatments, without a loss in the quality of service. There would be a corresponding increase in the number of people receiving treatment, creating vacancies to take on new patients from the waiting list.

While an appropriate lengthening in the return period is extremely important, even greater gains can be realised through eliminating other inefficiences. Forcing chiropodists to reconsider their patients afresh produced significant changes in the recommend treatment plans. The following table contrasts the previously existing patterns of care, with those recommended for the same patients during the research week (Table 24).

The simplest and most obvious of the improvements is the decrease in the percentage of patients on chiropody for life, from 91.2% to 80.7%. But if one remembers the large number of incomplete records which probably disguised still more routine maintenance, then the real drop approaches a fifth of all cases.

Intensive treatment plans

Behind this reduction lies a more complex change, however – the increased use of intensive treatment plans. For many patients, the optimum pattern of care is to bring their feet up to the best condition possible by a concerted course of treatment, followed by regular visits at longer intervals thereafter. Five of the treatment plans (numbers four, five, six, eight and nine) involve the use of intensive treatment first, followed by some other course of action. Summing up all these options, intensive treatment was being used on only 6.1% of patients. During the research week, however, chiropodists recommended it for 19.4% of the same people.

Intensive treatment first means different outcomes later. The chiropodists felt it would lead to a quadrupling of the patients who are cured and discharged. Expressed that way, in proportions, the improvement sounds large. In fact, the new recommendations represent only 10 people. The real gains will come not through discharging patients, but through caring for them differently following intensive treatment.

More substantial in volume terms is the number of patients whose need would be reduced to occasional treatment. They rise from 0.7% to 5.4% of cases. These are people who will be seen only twice a year or less.

Potential gain in using FCAs

The most important potential gain, however, lies in the use of FCAs. This treatment option had not been available to the chiropodists heretofore, since at the time of the research the district had no FCAs in post. But when given the chance to choose the most appropriate pattern of care for existing patients, the chiropodists recommended footcare assistance for 9.8% of all cases. In absolute numbers, across the district's community caseload, this means that 643 people could be treated by footcare assistants instead of chiropodists.

Table 24: Distribution of patients by treatment plans from existing records and chiropodists' recommendations

		Existing pattern of treatment %		*Chiropodists' recommendations* %	
1.	Advice appointment only	0.4	0.4	0.0	0.4 minimal treatment
2.	One treatment, then annual check up	0.0		0.4	
3.	One treatment, then discharge	0.0	0.4	0.2	1.7 curative treatment
4.	Intensive treatment, then discharge	0.4		1.5	
5.	Intensive treatment, then SOS only	0.7	0.7	2.2	5.4 occasional treatment
6.	Intensive treatment, then return intervals of 20 weeks or more	0.0		3.2	
7.	One treatment, then footcare assistant	0.0	0.0	6.3	9.8 footcare assistance
8.	Intensive treatment, then footcare assistant	0.0		3.5	
9.	Intensive treatment, then routine maintenance	5.0	91.2	9.1	80.7 chiropody for life
10.	Routine maintenance	86.2		71.6	
11.	No decision recorded	7.2		2.0	

This should be seen as the minimum estimate of possible transfers, however. As explained earlier, many chiropodists are wary of FCAs fearing that they will leave the NHS and set up as private chiropodists. Three-quarters of the chiropodists working for the district have private practice interests. That is to say, three-quarters of the chiropodists who participated in this study and who recommended the new treatment plans, might plausibly view footcare assistants as potential competitors. It may reasonably be assumed that they estimated the scope for employing them conservatively.

In contrast, many public sector chiropodists are enthusiastic supporters of the idea of footcare assistants, viewing them as essential to the growth and improved effectiveness of the profession, so long as they work under direct supervision from a state registered chiropodist. In principle, many of the chiropodists who work exclusively for the NHS believe in the maximum possible use of footcare assistants.

Therefore, it was decided that another analysis of the material should be undertaken. One of the authors is herself a practising chiropodist. Before undertaking any other processing of the data from the chiropodists' study, she read through the first five pages of each of the 540 interview-examination schedules. That is, she read all the information except the chiropodists' recommended treatment plans. Then, for each patient she chose a treatment plan, applying the values of those who positively affirm the use of FCAs. These recommendations were then compared with those of the other chiropodists.

This method has its own dangers. While the schedules may contain all relevant medical and chiropodial information, other factors, psychological ones for example, may have influenced the chiropodist's judgement, but which are not written on the forms. Alternatively, in any set of research schedules there are always omissions in the recording. Thus, it is possible that her judgements were made on partial or faulty information. Subject to this qualification, in comparing her treatment recommendations with those of the chiropodists, the authors were seeking to juxtapose maximum and minimum estimates of the potential change in patterns of care. The full results of all analyses are brought together in the following table:

Table 25: Distributions of patients by treatment plans

	Existing pattern of treatment %	Minimum change strategy %	Maximum change strategy %	Group	(subtotals) Existing / Min / Max
1. Advice appointment only	0.4	0.0	0.0	minimal treatment	0.4 / 0.4 / 0.0
2. One treatment, then annual check up	0.0	0.4	0.0		
3. One treatment, then discharge	0.0	0.2	0.7	curative treatment	0.4 / 1.7 / 1.7
4. Intensive treatment, then discharge	0.4	1.5	1.0		
5. Intensive treatment, then SOS only	0.7	2.2	1.9	occasional treatment	0.7 / 5.4 / 2.5
6. Intensive treatment, then return intervals of 20 weeks or more	0.0	3.2	0.6		
7. One treatment, then footcare assistant	0.0	6.3	13.3	footcare assistance	0.0 / 9.8 / 58.5
8. Intensive treatment, then footcare assistant	0.0	3.5	45.2		
9. Intensive treatment, then routine maintenance	5.0	9.1	24.8	chiropody for life	91.2 / 80.7 / 36.3
10. Routine maintenance	86.2	71.6	11.5		
11. No decision recorded	7.2	2.0	1.3		

The positive attitude towards footcare assistants makes a dramatic difference to treatment recommendations and all that would follow from them. Under the maximum change strategy, 58.5% of patients could be transferred to FCAs after some initial form of treatment, compared with 9.8% under the minimum strategy. Rather than creating 643 vacancies for treatment by chiropodists, there could be 3,844 openings, over four times the waiting list. The significance of this lies in the creation of new capacity, which is vital if we are ever to start reducing unmet need.

Under a realistic workload, the employment of one full-time footcare assistant would allow approximately 400 patients to be put on a nail cutting service. The chiropodists' recommendations therefore implied hiring the equivalent of one and a half FCAs. The maximum estimate would suggest work for almost ten such staff.

But footcare assistants do much more than just cut nails and give footwear advice. They provide a reception service, answer the telephone, prepare patients, instruments and surgeries, act as surgical assistants to chiropodists during more serious treatments, and clean up afterwards. And this describes only their present legitimate activity. One can easily foresee that, in addition to these hygiene tasks, they might take on an expanded health education role in the way that dental hygienists have done. They might also provide minor treatments with a scalpel as pedicurists already do.

Because so many chiropodists have viewed FCAs primarily as potential competitors in the provision of simple footcare in the private sector they have overlooked or underestimated the benefits to themselves of having footcare assistants to perform all these other tasks. One important gain is simply time. Without constant interruptions, the chiropodist has more time to discuss problems with patients, to make diagnoses, to think about options, and deliver treatments. There are also psychological benefits. The repetitive nature of the work becomes monotonous. Footcare assistants share these tasks. Instead of working in isolation, the chiropodist now has a colleague. And what is perhaps not so noble, but no less of a reward for that, the chiropodist gains in status through having an assistant. Under the experience of working with FCAs, chiropodists come to appreciate these other benefits.

In advancing these arguments, it is not necessary to bolster a case. There is proof. After the research had taken place, at the height of the political controversy over closure, the district hired a full-time footcare assistant. One might have anticipated resistance from some of the chiropodists. There was none. Quite the contrary, over time referrals to the FCA have steadily increased to the point where the district now employs three full-time assistants. Which is to say, the same chiropodists who made the original conservative recommendations are now using FCAs to twice the extent they anticipated and referrals are still rising.

Even more dramatic in quantitative terms is the difference between the minimum and maximum estimates in the use of intensive treatments. The chiropodists recommended that 19.4% of existing patients would benefit from such care. Under the maximum strategy, 73.4% of existing patients should receive these treatments.

Proving which of these divergent estimates is more nearly correct is, at the present time, both impossible and irrelevant. As indicated earlier in Chapter 12, intensive treatment clinics have been established for one morning each week at all the department's service sites. They were primarily intended for new patients, and have been consistently oversubscribed. Only a few existing patients who desperately need intensive treatment have been able to get access to them. All the district's chiropodists are requesting more time for this intensive work. But such treatment is very time-consuming and labour intensive for a small number of patients. It necessitates a reduction in the number of routine maintenance treatments that can be scheduled, without immediately producing a greater reduction in the demand for them. In the foreseeable future, the service will not be able to provide for intensive treatment for a quarter of existing patients, much less three quarters. But the significant and substantial point is that the district's chiropodists have taken to the opportunity for intensive treatment with enthusiasm. The ritual of routine maintenance is being broken.

Most important policy conclusion

The most important policy conclusion of all, however, lies in the comparison which shows the smallest quantitative difference. There is little to choose between the minimum and maximum estimates of the existing patients who can be discharged. There are very few in either case. Even the most enthusiastic reformers of the chiropody service will not be able to cure people at an advanced age, when their feet have been allowed to deteriorate throughout a working life. This is the finest testimony to the need to put primary emphasis in footcare on prevention.

Many distinct forms of inefficiency in the chiropody service have been pointed out in this chapter, but in order to make some global, overall estimate of the extent to which improvement was possible, one final comparison of the three analyses, was made.

All the many complex treatment recommendations were simplified into three possible outcomes. Would the patients, under the new recommendations, receive more treatment, less treatment, or the same amount of treatment as they were receiving before? For example, if the patient is already receiving the optimum treatment plan, there will be no difference in the amount of treatment given. But if the patient is currently receiving routine maintenance, a recommendation for intensive treatment followed by footcare would lead not only to more appropriate, but also to less treatment – a simultaneous gain in organisational efficiency and individual care.

The new recommendations should represent considered opinions on the best course of treatment for the patient. The analysis of records represents the present state of affairs. The difference between the two is a measure of potential inefficiency and potential improvement, both in the care of the patient and the operation of the service. The differences between the existing pattern of care and the minimum and maximum change strategies are summarised below.

Table 26: Volume of treatment under different plans

	Minimum change strategy	Maximum change strategy
Less treatments than existing pattern	33.3%	82.6%
Equal number of treatments as existing pattern	57.0%	9.4%
More treatments than existing pattern	2.1%	0.8%
Missing data so comparison impossible	7.6%	7.2%

When records are taken away from them, in only 57% of the cases do chiropodists recommend the same treatment as the patient had been receiving before. This suggests, *prima facie*, that chiropodists are often just perpetuating the previous pattern of care. And 'copying-on' usually means providing more treatments than necessary. At the very minimum, a third of patients were receiving chiropody too often. Probably, most were having too much.

Clearly, a fresh reconsideration of patients' problems not only means better care, it means less treatment as well. That approach, applied to the service as a whole, would create sufficient new capacity to start doing something about unmet need.

Considerable inefficiency

The analysis so far revealed considerable inefficiency: too many routine maintenance treatments, excessively frequent appointments, expensive chiropodists doing sub-chiropodial work. And all this has been found in what is thought to be one of the better chiropody departments in the NHS. Even the maximum estimates for this district may underestimate the inefficiency prevailing in some other parts of the country.

The common factor underlying all the problems described in this section is that they are caused by chiropodists themselves, and therefore solvable within the service itself. The problems described here may be seen, in part, as the outcome of two contrasting perspectives and interests, that of the individual chiropodist who has to treat the patients, and that of the chiropody manager who has to organise the district's service. Both need to change.

Seen from the perspective of the clinical chiropodist, who more often than not is a part-timer doing sessions for the NHS, this 'inefficiency' is not so irrational. Because of the priority group system, he deals almost exclusively with elderly patients whose problems are so far advanced that practically all attempts at cure are fruitless. If he does make an intensive effort to improve a patient's condition and reduce the frequency of visits, his immediate reward is to receive off the waiting list another elderly patient whose feet are in worse condition. In any case, providing long sessions of intensive treatment is difficult, because the administrative system books in a standard number of people for standard time periods. If, within these constraints, he schedules his patients for frequent palliative treatments, at least this means there is less deterioration and less discomfort between visits, and therefore less work for him at each visit. In theory, this might mean he could give more treatments each day. But then 'custom and practice' within chiropody frequently dictates that the standard workload for the standard three-hour clinical session is eight patients. So he finishes early instead. If he recognises, as many do, that some of his patients do not really need his skills at all, but could be treated quite adequately by a footcare assistant, there is still none in post to refer them to. Seen from his perspective then, what has been described as 'inefficiency' may also be just a rational response to the system of which he finds himself temporarily a part. Some chiropodists may, of course, be genuinely apathetic. But a rational man might act in much the same way.

The task of management is not just to exhort people to work more efficiently, but to make it possible for them to do so. In several ways the administrative system was blocking chiropodists from doing as good a job as they wanted to do. There have been many changes in the district's management system (see Chapter 23, Table 34). The two changes relevant here have been the employment of footcare assistants and the organisation of intensive care clinics. Once established, chiropodists have made much more use of these options than either they or the managers thought they would. Once the service was reorganised to allow chiropodists to practice better chiropody, they did so. And as part of the new spirit, the standard workload per session has recently been renegotiated so that the chiropodists are fully occupied for the whole session.

In a service with such an overhang of unmet need, self-congratulation would be premature. But some of the inefficiences this research discovered are being eliminated, some of the potential gains are being realised. In the world of chiropody at least, breaking the mould is possible.

18 Expansion: new roles, new resources

If we step back from the details of current footcare provision, and look at the broad pattern of service, we see a curious and costly imbalance. Footcare in the NHS today is provided by a number of highly skilled professionals – district nurses, general practitioners, hospital doctors, chiropodists, surgeons and physiotherapists. All undergo long training and are, relatively at least, well paid. There are comparatively few basic carers, providing simple inexpensive treatments for simple foot problems.

Yet many foot problems are simple. The research has documented a large volume of need for basic foot hygiene and simple palliative treatments of a routine, repeated kind. Much of this work could be carried out, under supervision, by less highly qualified personnel. And the study has repeatedly pointed out omissions, other important work that the chiropody service cannot now undertake because of the load of treatments – initial screening programmes and educational/advisory services on footwear and footcare. Many people could undertake such activity, with only a modest specialist training in footcare.

In the absence of an adequate supply of people at the basic care level, all foot treatment, even the most elementary, is now provided by chiropodists – a group which spends three years full-time in training, then spends much of its time at work providing basic foot hygiene – what was earlier described as the sub-chiropodial part of the footcare spectrum. This is a very expensive way to cut peoples' toenails. Of all the mismatches of problems to personnel in footcare, this is the most costly. Using surgeons to remove ingrown toenails is more expensive per procedure, but using chiropodists for foot hygiene is much more widespread. This is mass, rather than élite, inefficiency.

There is also the consequential problem: whenever chiropodists are doing sub-chiropodial work, they are not doing chiropodial work and people with serious foot problems go untreated. Yet the research repeatedly demonstrated a substantial requirement for intensive treatment both among existing patients and among those with unmet needs. The waiting list study documented the need for urgent treatment. All of this is work that can only be undertaken by fully trained chiropodists. Much of it is not being done, because they are doing foot hygiene instead.

In sum, the research found substantial unmet need for both highly skilled chiropody and elementary footcare. This is not surprising. The service is so short of resources one would expect to find unmet needs at all levels of the footcare spectrum. But the way footcare provision is currently organised, the greatest shortage is not at the top of the skill hierarchy, but at the bottom. We need to develop new roles and recruit new people for sub-chiropodial care.

To start by dealing with the shortage at the bottom is ironically also the best way to deal with the shortage at the top. The quickest way to inject more skilled people into the chiropody service is by releasing already trained chiropodists from their sub-chiropodial work. We certainly need to train more chiropodists, but this is a long and expensive process, so the growth in numbers is slow. Employing new staff at basic care grades, will have a greater effect, more quickly and less expensively. It deals with both ends of the problem simultaneously.

We need therefore to develop substantial new sources of sub-chiropodial manpower. But is this a practical proposition? Can we find people in sufficient numbers to undertake these new roles? Can we provide even the limited training they need without new finance? And can we afford to employ them once they are trained? Can we do the economically impossible – vastly increase a service without increasing expenditure? In a word, yes.

Footcare assistants (FCAs)

The potential of FCAs, both in the provision of care and in health education, was described in the last chapter. It was made clear that their use should be expanded to the maximum extent possible subject to direct supervision by a chiropodist. Here the economic aspect of that expansion is considered.

Training for sub-chiropodial care is much less time-consuming than for chiropody (a matter of weeks rather than years) and much less costly (hundreds of pounds not thousands). Within the NHS, FCAs are also less expensive to employ. At present, they provide only nail cutting and education, but an expansion of their role would mean we could treat a substantial proportion of the service's patients at a lower cost per patient. This gain in efficiency would enable more people to be taken on.

To make it absolutely clear what is being proposed: it is suggested that FCAs should be used to release chiropodists to deal with more serious cases. This is not a proposal for cheap substitution, for sacking chiropodists and taking on FCAs instead. Nor is there the faintest likelihood that this would happen in practice. To see why, one must appreciate the quite extraordinary labour market in chiropody.

State registered chiropodists are in extremely short supply. They have no problem finding work – full or part-time, in any part of the country they choose, in private practice or the public sector or any combination of the two. The principal buyer, the NHS, only employs state registered chiropodists. Most health districts cannot find enough to fill their existing establishments/budgets. The majority do not even receive any applications when they advertise posts. The problem is not just the general shortage. The priority group system means that NHS chiropody involves a great deal of low-skill and repetitive work, exclusively with elderly people. Some chiropodists prefer a more varied workload elsewhere.

What most district chiropody services must do to cover the gap in their staffing, is to buy-in part-timers from the outside to do clinical sessions. In some health districts there is only one full-time chiropodist. All the rest are 'sessionals', paid on a complex, graduated scale depending on the number of hours they work. The highest rate is paid for the first four sessions or 12 hours a week, so this is what most sessionals work. On an hourly basis, this rate is 50% above that paid to an equivalent chiropodist in the NHS, even after including all the extra employer contributions. This is the premium the NHS is paying to attract part-time staff. This is a costly way to provide chiropody. And it is made absurdly more expensive when these high-priced sessionals spend so much of their time doing sub-chiropodial work.

The proposal is to give as much of this sub-chiropodial work as possible to footcare assistants, to enable chiropody services to reduce the number of sessions they fill with part-timers from the outside. There is no worry that the sessionals thereby released will become unemployed. In the current state of excess demand for footcare, there is more than ample work for a state registered chiropodist in the private sector.

Ironically, however, employing more FCAs will help the NHS to employ more registered chiropodists as well. If much of the routine, low-skill, palliative work is taken over by footcare assistants, this will change the nature of the job for chiropodists. Chiropody within the NHS will become a higher-skill, more challenging, and therefore more attractive task. In fact, this is just what has happened in the research district. At the same time as it gradually moved to employing three footcare assistants, it has also increased its full-time registered chiropodists from five to ten.

By reducing the volume of part-time work paid at premium rates, the NHS will be able, within the same budget, to hire both footcare assistants and more state registered chiropodists, thereby increasing the capacity of the service. In sum, it is possible to expand the service without raising expenditure.

However, the much more conventional economics of the private sector may determine those of the public. It appears, from evidence presented in Chapter 21, that there is a substantial volume of basic foot hygiene and low-skill work being done by private chiropodists in response to public demand. They could employ footcare assistants to do it, but apparently relatively few do. They fear that these assistants would soon leave and set up as rivals. Under current regulations there is nothing to stop this.

These anxieties about competition are increased by the prospect of introducing numbers of footcare assistants into the NHS, some of whom would sooner or later leave the public sector and establish private practices themselves. Two have done so already. The fear of competition is therefore realistic.

State registered chiropodists in the private sector could influence the decision about footcare assistants within the NHS because many district chiropody services are utterly dependent on sessional and contract work by registered chiropodists in private practice. In making these points private chiropody is neither being attacked or supported; the authors are simply acknowledging that private registered chiropodists have it in their power to block the reform advocated, and all the benefits which flow from it. The successful introduction of FCAs will depend, in part, on coming to some kind of agreement with them. This points again to the need for the DHSS to take active measures to break the stalemate over the linked issues of footcare and closure. Realising the economies will depend on political initiative.

Nurses

Nurses are already health professionals trained far above the level needed for sub-chiropodial footcare. But few have had specialist instruction in the problems of the foot and hence give them no particular emphasis in the course of their work. All this is normal and understandable.

But is so happens that three types of nurses work in roles where they could make an important contribution to footcare, school nurses, district nurses and health visitors. Between them they have contacts with two groups which, for different reasons, are important if we are ever going to improve foot health, the young and the old. The nurses provide various mixtures of inspection, advice and treatment. Footcare figures little in their activity and, of course, they already have more than enough commitments. But with a modest investment in training, no increase in current expenditure, and only a small addition to their workload, they could help with the prevention, detection and treatment of foot problems.

School nurses

The school nurses' work at a critical moment in the emergence of foot problems has already been described, and the potential for improved screening and education. Chiropodists know that such preventive work with schoolchildren is vital to the future of foot health and the footcare services. But being realistic, faced with their clinical load, they know they will never be able to undertake such work on anything like the scale needed. Treatment forces out prevention. School nurses are thus potentially a large and essential new labour resource for footcare. And all that is necessary to develop it is to help them to do their present job better.

District nurses

Peripatetic treatment in the community is provided by district nurses, especially for elderly people. At present they do only a little footcare, but they do sometimes wash old people's feet as part of their general work. With a little extra training they could do nail cutting and simple palliative treatments. While this sounds a modest task, its economic significance is large. The elderly people whom district nurses treat are often the same people who require expensive domiciliary visits from chiropodists. At the same time, the nurses could inspect the feet for the development of more serious problems which require referral for specialist chiropody. Finally, they are in a good position to give advice on that often overlooked source of foot problems to the housebound elderly, indoor footwear. That particular subject will be returned to in Chapter 20. The point here is that district nurses could become a cost-effective additional source of treatment for a particularly vulnerable section of the group that requires the most footcare.

Health visitors

As the final pages of this book were being written a four-month old baby was brought to the district chiropody service with an in-grown toenail. It was apparently caused by pressure from a stretch, all-in-one baby suit. The damage to children's feet can begin long before they reach their first school health inspection. Health visitors already do systematic educational work with mothers and young children. Amidst all the other information to be conveyed, relatively little is done on foot health. All that is really required is to raise health visitor's awareness and specialist knowledge of foot problems, so that these receive a higher priority in their work. They are ideally placed to give advice on footcare and footwear. And footwear, as the example makes clear, includes hose as well as shoes.

Voluntary organisations

In recent years there has been a proliferation of 'nail cutting services' run by voluntary organisations for vulnerable groups in society, usually elderly and handicapped people. In establishing these services, the voluntary agencies have been responding to a definite need, as the research confirms. Groups which work with elderly people have persistently appealed for statutory agencies to provide more of this service. But the general shortage of chiropodists and the already long waiting lists have meant that district chiropody services could seldom respond on the scale demanded. Some voluntary groups have therefore taken the initiative and established nail cutting services themselves. This is an understandable response. Voluntary organisations have frequently filled in gaps or supplemented the statutory services and this role has increased markedly since the 1960s. Exactly how many voluntary groups have moved into this work is not known, but a research project on the subject has just begun.

Chiropodists have frequently opposed these developments. This, too, is an understandable response. Voluntary organisations commonly underestimate the complexity of apparently simple nail cutting and the dangers introduced by other medical conditions. Some schemes are also undermanaged, with little or no training for the volunteer nail cutters and inadequate supervision of their work. This is not always the case. Sometimes voluntary groups have worked in collaboration with the NHS, where registered chiropodists screen patients and deal with serious cases, while the volunteers cut nails. But there are enough ill-organised schemes to cause genuine anxiety.

Thus both sides are behaving reasonably. But neither is achieving what it would like. The clients of the voluntary organisations are receiving a service that is more risky and less good than it might be. And chiropodists' opposition verges on the counterproductive. In the voluntary sector, registered chiropodists have no power to determine what decisions are taken. Voluntary groups can and do turn to non-registered chiropodists or other health professionals to establish their schemes. A substantial new development is taking place in chiropody's area of expertise, but almost completely outside the profession's influence.

Let us set this voluntary development in context. There is a great volume of need for basic foot hygiene of the type that could be provided adequately by volunteers, if they were properly trained and supervised. Chiropodists know this need exists because they spend so much of their time meeting it under the existing organisation of NHS chiropody. Yet there is no prospect that the NHS will ever be able to cope with this blocked excess demand. In the name of maintaining high standards of care, many will never receive any care at all.

Against this background, voluntary organisations represent a major new labour resource for footcare. Potentially, they could make a substantial contribution to expanding services in precisely that area where the shortage is greatest, sub-chiropodial work. This opportunity must be positively developed as energetically as possible. This will require changed attitudes and more co-operative behaviour from both sides.

The voluntary organisations must recognise that footcare, even nail cutting, is complicated. They must involve fully-qualified chiropodists first in the screening of potential patients and then in supervising the work that is done by the volunteers. They must recognise the need to train their volunteers not only in nail cutting techniques, but in recognising problems which must be referred.

Chiropodists, in turn, must recognise what an opportunity this voluntary initiative represents for them and for their patients. Instead of objecting from the outside that the schemes are, or may be, improperly run, they must ensure from the inside that they operate correctly. This means a positive engagement with voluntary organisations to establish, organise and develop nail cutting services on a local basis. It means establishing training programmes and assuming responsibility for supervising the work.

Expansion is possible. It is feasible to obtain new resources for the chronically under-resourced footcare services. But this entails rethinking how we provide footcare. It involves more than just an acceptance of change; it requires a positive engagement to shape change. New roles will have to be developed, new training programmes established, new relationships built with outside organisations. It will not happen easily or quickly and it will demand more than a co-operative spirit. In some areas there will have to be hard political negotiations, compromises, reallocation of resources, and a redefinition of prerogatives, for chiropodists and for everyone else involved in footcare.

But the alternative is an increasingly overloaded service. Setting the changing demography of the country against the medium-term prospects for chiropodial manpower, the authors can only forecast a stagnation of supply in the face of increasing demand, a growing imbalance between need and provision. Developing new sub-chiropodial roles in large numbers is the most cost-effective way to expand the provision of footcare in Britain today. For practical purposes, it is the only way we will ever make serious inroads into the problem of unmet need.

19 Conclusion: inefficiency is hopeful

The second part of this research has indicated, with varying degrees of thoroughness, considerable inefficiency among all the major providers of footcare in Britain today. This is extremely hopeful.

At least inefficiency indicates that there is the possibility of improvement, potential to expand the capacity of the footcare services within existing financial constraints. Realising that potential by eliminating that inefficiency will be difficult, of course. But better matching of problems to personnel will make it possible to deal with the whole range of foot conditions more cheaply, enabling chiropodists to take on more patients within the same budget. Better planning of treatment will reduce the quantity of individual care while raising its quality, thereby releasing new capacity to start reducing the backlog of need.

To these gains through eliminating inefficiency, we may add the other potential gains indicated in the second part of the research, new sources of manpower for basic footcare. In these new resources lie not only the possibility of increasing treatment capacity, but the beginnings of a move into preventive footcare.

It would be premature to estimate how much difference these changes could make, premature to make any promises of improvement. The concrete steps that need to be taken by all the many people involved in footcare are set out in detail in the final policy and practice section. But to sum up the point of the research to this stage with an ironic conclusion: things are so bad there is hope. The first two sections of this book have demonstrated problems with footcare on a greater scale than anyone has heretofore suggested. This demonstration has not been intended as criticism, in a destructive sense. It has been intended to point out specific areas for improvement.

Part IV

Footwear and Footcare

20 'Shoes can damage your health'

Although the intrinsic strength and individual structure of each foot make the chance of foot problems more or less probable, there is little doubt that footwear (hose as well as shoes) plays an important part. Much emphasis is therefore put on footwear for the maintenance of foot health. A badly fitted shoe can produce corns and callouses in a foot that is normal when bare. Footwear may not cause curly toes, but can produce corns on the dorsal (upper) surface and prevent the toes from straightening naturally. And inadequate footwear can exacerbate many conditions.

What then is adequate footwear? A basic definition is footwear which does not restrict the natural function of the foot and which gives adequate protection from climate and local environment. Thus it may range from a basic sole with thongs to attach it to the foot, through to specialist safety shoes. If the shoe does not enclose the foot, the foot must not overhang the sole, and foot and shoe must remain in a proper relationship when the foot is in motion.

For closed-in shoes, which encase the toes, fitting is far more complex. The major points are listed below.

1. *LENGTH*. It must be long enough to accommodate the foot with ½in (¾in in children) gap between the longest toe and the end of the shoe when standing. This allows the toes room to move.
2. *WIDTH*. It must be wide enough to allow the toes to rest on the insole, without being cramped together and without causing the uppers to bulge out sideways.
3. *DEPTH*. The front of the shoe must be deep enough so that the uppers do not press on the toes, as this will cause corns or the toenails to impinge on the flesh causing pain and/or damage to the nail itself.

4. *FASTENING.* If the shoe is fitted to meet the requirements above, it will also need to have an adjustable fastening across the instep, so the foot and shoe remain in the same relationship whilst the foot is moving. Otherwise, the foot will slide forward in the shoe, causing the toes to be cramped and the heel of the shoe to slip off.

5. *HEELS.* Other important features of the shoe are its heel height, 1½in being the maximum for adults if overloading of the forefoot is not to take place. The area of the heel base is also important; the larger it is, the more stable a base it provides for walking.

It is not only shoes which can cause damage – tight hose can also do so. Very small babies may only have their feet uncovered whilst being bathed or changed. Knitted bootees, which used to be the fashion, were sometimes criticised for restricting freedom of foot movement but had the advantage that the baby frequently managed to get them off. Unfortunately the present all-in-one stretch suits include 'feet' as part of the garment. These cannot be wiggled off, and the force exerted by the garment is borne by the toes. Stretch socks may also constrict the toes, if fitted too small; they may also contribute to the illusion that tight shoes fit, because the socks are already cramping the toes.

Whilst the importance of having the feet measured and shoes fitted at every purchase cannot be stressed too much, the principles which have been outlined here are the ones which should be applied if a purchase has to be made without the help of a properly trained shoe fitter.

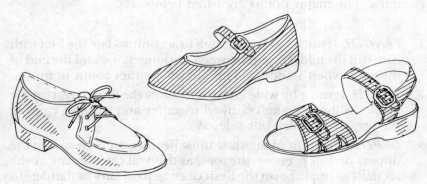

Fig. 4: Acceptable styles

All the investigations into need for footcare recorded the type of footwear usually worn. In children, footwear can play a part in damaging young feet, whilst in the older age groups, it can and does cause or exacerbate problems. Moreover, old or sloppy footwear can lead to accidents. The main points related to each population group will now be considered in turn.

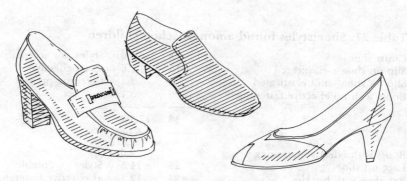

Fig. 5: Unacceptable styles

Children's footwear

Only 29% of the children had shoes that met the standard outlined above. The remarks about footwear in this chapter thus relate only to shoes because the school nurses' timetable made it impossible to look at hose. Children often undressed outside the room; many had to be sent back for their shoes. This may explain why school nurses do not refer for footwear advice – they don't actually see the child in shoes.

The vast majority of children were in danger of developing toe deformities due to wearing ill-fitting shoes. A dramatic example of the damage which can be done by constricting the feet was the now illegal practice of foot binding in China. The feet were bound tightly in childhood when the skeleton of the foot is mostly cartilage. This prevented the growth as the bone developed during childhood and adolescence and, by about the age of 20, the feet were fully ossified at 3 to 4 inches in length, so that the woman had to be carried everywhere. The bound feet were thus set to remain that size for life. In a less extreme way, badly fitted footwear can do the same today.

Shoe style

Nine broad categories of footwear were found amongst the children. None of the schools in the survey prescribed uniform shoe styles or, apparently, restricted the type of shoe worn. It is ironic that there is no school policy for the one piece of clothing which can do actual harm.

Table 27: Shoe styles found amongst schoolchildren

Court shoe	8	4.0	Styles not acceptable
Slip-on shoe – elasticated	15	7.6	as no effective
Slip-on shoe – not elasticated	6	3.1	fastening present
Boots with no effective fastening	6	3.1	
	35	17.8%	
Boots with effective fastening	4	2.0	
Lace-up shoe	28	14.3	Styles acceptable
Bar shoe with buckle	25	12.8	as effective fastening
Sandals	21	10.7	present
Plimsolls/trainers (with laces)	83	42.3	
	161	82.1%	
TOTAL	196	100%	

Four of the styles, worn by 17.8% of the children, were unacceptable because they simply slipped onto the foot or had elastic gussets. Elastic is not strong enough to hold the foot steady in the shoe. Whilst style is of interest, an acceptable style is no guarantee of the shoe being an adequate fit.

Shoe fitting

Of the children whose footwear was of an acceptable style, 104 had shoes which did not fit, a further 53% of the total. Thus, of the total 196 children whose footwear styles were recorded, only 29.2% had shoes which actually fitted. Thus more than two thirds of the children sampled were at risk of foot deformity accelerated or caused by their footwear. A much respected chiropodist once expressed the wish that children could be blessed with feet that hurt when their footwear becomes too small – it would save a lot of misery later in life, when the effects of poorly fitted footwear become apparent.

Table 28 shows the reasons why shoes did not fit, using the criteria in the fitting standard used above.

Table 28: Reasons why children's shoes did not fit

Length inadequate	122
Width inadequate	42
Depth of toe box inadequate	35
No fastening present	35
Heel too high	18
Heel base area inadequate	6

The fact that inadequate length was the overwhelming reason for shoes not fitting serves to emphasise that children outgrow their shoes before wearing them out, or indeed have shoes bought which are too short already. Because children's feet are so rarely painful, even in shoes which are too small, it is all too easy for even the most caring adult to overlook the necessity for new shoes. The danger is an insidious one – unnoticed until too late.

If only 29% had adequately fitting shoes, which styles were these? Thirty-five children were wearing plimsolls or training shoes. Trainers were popular, especially with boys. They have three advantages: they have laces, they wear out quickly and they can be bought cheaply. The laces usually start from a point quite near the toes, allowing adjustment to fit correctly. Whilst badly fitting trainers may be as harmful as badly fitting shoes, they will wear out and be replaced more often. This at least allows the chance for a larger size to be purchased. More durable leather shoes, especially if well made, will both cost more and last much longer and there is therefore a great danger that they will be outgrown before they are outworn. Durability is not necessarily a virtue in children's shoes.

Laced shoes are particularly good as they can be adjusted to each foot exactly, no pair of feet ever being exactly the same shape or size. It appeared that trainers were the only lace-ups which were fashionable, and therefore being chosen. Certainly for girls it is difficult to buy a lace-up which would be seen as fashionable and acceptable. Ten children wore lace-ups other than trainers.

The next best thing to laces are shoes which buckle. Buckles must not be on elastic because under strain the foot will slide in the shoe. Straps and buckles cannot be adjusted as finely as laces, but it is usually possible to fasten the shoe to the foot adequately. Eleven children had buckled shoes.

The remaining child was wearing wooden sandals with a strap across the base of the toes. Whilst they may not have been wise from a safety aspect they fitted properly and she walked easily and naturally in them. The long term effects, if any, of such footwear are unknown.

Of the children whose shoes fitted, 68% were boys and 32% were girls. This may reflect the fact that most shoes made for boys and men are quite close in shape to the human foot – this is certainly untrue of women's shoes which are generally long and slender, whereas the foot is somewhat triangular. This may also partially explain why far more women have foot problems than men. Even for women who want a shoe which fastens and fits, it may be difficult to find something in an acceptable price range.

Purchase points

The researchers were interested not only in the fit of the children's shoes, but also in who was involved in their purchase. Most of the children were happy to say who chose the shoes and where they were bought. This was one area of the examination where lack of privacy was a positive help as the children frequently discussed the subject amongst themselves whilst waiting. As there was no way of checking that the answers given by the children were accurate, the results in this section can only be suggestive of the pattern of shoe purchase. It is a subject which should be pursued at a later date, as shoe purchase is both difficult and important for good foot health.

Of the total sample 117 (57%) said that they accompanied their parent(s) or another adult to the shop to purchase the shoes which were being worn. It is always advisable to take the child to the shop when purchasing footwear so that the shoes can be tried on, even if no trained shoe fitter is available. Some 20 children (9.8%) had their shoes brought home for them, a proportion of whom told us that this was because their mother was at work and bought them in her lunch hour. But this does not give the whole explanation as shoe shops are open on Saturdays. Only one child of the total sample was wearing shoes which had been handed down from another child. These in fact fitted, although the wear marks on the soles showed the chiropodist instantly that they had been passed on. Shoes should not be passed from child to child because, if they are at all worn, the shoes may cause the second wearer to walk badly or they may not fit properly. Five children reported that they bought their shoes alone, but this information may be the result of bragging in front of other children. Thirty children said that sometimes they went to the shop and sometimes the shoes were brought home – not all could remember for the shoes being worn and thus a 'mixed' pattern of purchase was recorded. One child went to the shops with a sibling under 18.

The total sample was divided according to who was involved in the shoe purchase, and whether or not the shoes fitted. It was not known if any of the children had their feet measured, but few traditional shoes were seen. The two groups were compared in order to see if there as any significant difference. In fact, there was none. The proportions of each group (not fitting versus fitting) were very similar, although the numbers in the two groups were very different. One would have expected that more of the children with fitting shoes would have gone to the shop with a parent. The results are shown in the table below:

Table 29: People involved in shoe purchase

	Shoes did not fit		Shoes fitted	
Adult with child	83	66%	34	70%
Adult without child	16	12%	2	4%
Child alone	3	2%	4	8%
Shoes passed down	0	0%	1	2%
Other	24	19%	7	14%
	126	99%	48	98%

This would suggest that the purchasing of shoes which fitted was largely by accident. The reasons for this are unknown and merit further investigation. It is possible to suggest some of the reasons. First, in the research district there are few shops with a shoe fitting service. Only one is listed in the Children's Foot Health Register – 'a guide to shops which stock children's shoes in width fittings and where trained staff will measure both feet and fit the shoes at the time of sale'. Also, many shoe shops are small, local businesses, probably supplied by the several small shoe factories within the district. Another factor may be that shoes which come in width fittings and half sizes are generally more expensive than shoes made in a single width, and whole sizes only, not simply because of increased production costs but because they are made of leather, not of cheap plastic. No attempt was made to gauge the socio-economic class of the children, but the research district is one of the most deprived areas in Britain.

If the footwear and standard of fitting is at all representative, a large number of children are at risk.

The next part of this chapter illustrates that the situation is little better where elderly people are concerned.

Elderly people

In elderly people, whilst well-fitting shoes will not undo the ravages of time, they can sometimes prevent the formation of corns or callosities simply because they do not interfere with foot function any more than absolutely necessary. Well fitted shoes also enable professional treatment to be more effective, by allowing room for padding or corrective devices. Badly fitted shoes may not only cause problems and prevent their cure, but may also contribute to a reduction in mobility due to feelings of instability of balance.

In all three studies which involved elderly people, that is the waiting list, those currently receiving chiropody treatment and the unmet need study, the type of shoes worn both inside the house and outside was investigated.

Over half, 57%, said that they normally wore shoe styles which were considered by chiropodists as unacceptable (due to lack of a fastening). This figure gives the impression that just under half the elderly population are choosing and wearing shoes which have the potential to fit properly. However, it was felt that many older people might not actually spend much time in their outdoor shoes.

When the time factor is introduced, the results are dramatically different.

Table 30: Shoe styles worn by elderly people

	Current Patient Study	Waiting List Study	Unmet Need Study	TOTAL	
Acceptable styles worn for 8 hours or more	108	22	7	137	15%
Unacceptable styles worn for majority of day	394	348	25	767	85%
TOTAL	502	370	32	904	100%

Thus, whilst 43% of elderly people choose acceptable shoes for outdoor wear, only 15% actually wear them for the greater part of the day. Most elderly people spend most of their time in slippers, or slip-on shoes.

This has great implications for people's foot health. Whilst shoes are not responsible alone for foot trouble, they do play a role and it would appear that most people are not wearing a sensible shoe for most of the time. It is NOT suggested that people should never wear unacceptable styles but simply that their use should be kept to a minimum. One immediate way in which to start to remedy the situation is education of the public. Chiropodists, whilst giving treatment, are ideally placed to give advice and information regarding footwear to their patients, and it would be reasonable to expect people receiving treatment to have more suitable footwear choices. However, the table shows that the differences between elderly people on the waiting list, and those receiving treatment is very small, and may be due to chance, and the fact that one study was done in late winter and the other in late spring. However, it would appear that chiropodists have little influence on footwear choice.

As well as recording the actual style and duration of wearing, some attempts were made to ascertain people's attitudes to footwear, ie. whether they thought their footwear had any influence on their feet, and if a change of style would help them. The information collected here is open to question as the respondents may have given the answer which they thought the interviewer wanted, especially those who knew or guessed the interviewer to be a chiropodist. However, in none of the studies did recognition of the fact that footwear might affect the feet exceed 27% of the total answers received.

Over half of these positive answers came from people wearing acceptable shoe styles. It would appear that they have found, by experience or through advice taken, that shoes which fasten are better for them. But they are a small minority.

For some elderly people, a change of style may be physically impossible, due to an inability to cope with conventional laces and buckles, but this problem may often be overcome by use of 'touch and close' fastenings, one-handed lacing or use of zip fasteners. (See *Footcare and footwear for disabled children; Footwear and footcare for adults* and *Footwear for problem feet*). Many more may not understand the relationship between foot and shoe. Some may not want to understand! Footwear advice is not always welcome and it is well known to chiropodists that some patients come in shoes which they wear only to avoid repeat advice, which they do not wish to take.

Policy implications

The policy implications from these studies of footwear may be grouped under (i) education and (ii) shoe design and fitting.

Education

Foot health education is relevant to all age groups. Whilst babies and small children cannot be responsible for their own foot health, they are a vulnerable group; expectant mothers and parents should therefore be helped to an awareness of the importance of their children's feet. In schools, foot health should be part of the curriculum. It is inevitable that other health subjects such as smoking and sex education will take precedence, but foot health can be brought into other subject areas, such as sport, art, history or fashion/design. Schools could also encourage foot health awareness by simple rules regarding footwear, insisting, for example, that shoes have a fastening across the instep and flat heels. This would not solve the fitting problem, but would at least make parents aware of two basic precepts, without imposing a price burden on the less affluent.

If foot damage from footwear could be minimised up to the age of 18, more adults would reach retirement age with comfortable feet than at present. For some, the habit of wearing shoes with fastening whilst at school, would persist at work, although fashion shoes would undoubtedly be worn at other times. The time factor for potential damage would, however, be reduced. In the elderly groups, there is an obvious need for education on the effect which footwear has on feet, regardless of the condition of those feet.

One problem, not covered by the research but which is familiar to anyone who tries to advise on footwear is the common belief that 'good = expensive'. Whilst this may be true, it is equally possible to spend large sums of money on shoes with no fastenings which are therefore going to be 'bad' for the feet. However, preaching the gospel of leather, width-fitting shoes may be counter-productive if people feel that this type of shoe is beyond their means. It may prove that an educative campaign based on style might be of more practical benefit. Manufacturers and health educators (of all disciplines) could then put out the same message: 'It's not the price that counts, but the fit'. The idea that a fastening is a pre-requisite to any style of shoe which can be fitted properly needs to be made obvious to the public, backed up with other information on how to buy shoes which fit.

This leads on to the other policy issue: practicality. It is all very well to educate people, but, unless the choice of footwear is available at a reasonable price, no real good will be achieved.

Shoe design and fitting

Some makes of children's shoes come in half sizes and width fittings. Excellent as they are, they are also expensive when it is remembered that they are soon outgrown (see the National Consumer Council's *Bad fit, bad feet*). Many more children's shoes come in full sizes and one width only. Short of legal restrictions on their manufacture/import, they are not going to disappear from shops, and without financial penalties to increase the price, many parents will opt for these cheaper shoes, either from choice or due to low incomes. The problem must therefore be tackled differently. A start could be made by **all** shoe retail staff having a basic training in shoe fitting for children. Many have trained staff (the Children's Foot Health Register is one source of information), but children's shoes can be bought off the shelf. Some retailers will not sell shoes if the child isn't present; this should be encouraged.

Elderly people are a considerable consumer group. Whilst they may have a lower income, they do represent some 15% of the total population of the UK. They could, if motivated, provide a considerable pressure group for more shoes suited to their frequently misshapen feet. Such shoes are often expensive and the general image presented is seen as frumpy, old fashioned or 'granny style', even by older people themselves. If the demand for wide fitting, fastening shoes were sufficiently visible, manufacturers would produce more fashionable styles.

Again, retailers could be encouraged to provide more fitting services. Members of the Society of Shoe Fitters provide such services in many shops but there simply are not enough of them.

Lastly, a revolution in the slipper market is needed. It is very difficult to purchase slippers which fasten, but it is surely not beyond the realms of possibility to design, manufacture and sell a soft, possibly fleecy-lined shoe, with a slip-resistant sole which won't break up, and a fastening. This does not have to be laces or buckles – 'touch and close' fastenings, as used on clothes and running shoes, would be quite satisfactory.

21 The changing role of chiropody

Earlier the ambiguity surrounding chiropody and how it affected relations with patients and with other health professionals was described. But chiropodists themselves differ on the subject. Some differing conceptions are to be expected, between the registered and the non-registered, for example, or between those working in the NHS and those in private practice. The situation has been further complicated in recent years by advances in the skill and training of chiropodists. Because chiropody is so significant in the range of footcare services, a special investigation was made of chiropodists' views on the changing role of chiropody.

Chiropodists were sent a postal questionnaire – a three page document requiring two sheets to be completed and returned. The top sheet was an introduction to the concept that footcare went beyond the realm of chiropody, including areas of both sub-chiropody and supra-chiropody. The idea of the footcare spectrum was presented with nail cutting and basic hygiene at one end (ie. that which most adults do for themselves) with a variety of skills and conditions in the middle and major surgery at the other end (see Table 4 page 19). 'Chiropody' obviously falls somewhere between, but the problem is 'where'? The intention was that, by completing the questionnaire, the chiropodists would indicate where they would draw the boundaries of their scope of practice. Additionally, the questionnaire asked for details of the type(s) of employment currently being undertaken and the year they commenced practice.

Rather than straight questions, the two sheets to be completed consisted of descriptions of 14 hypothetical patients, about whom the chiropodists had to make a decision on future treatment. For each patient there was a description-diagnosis of (i) the foot condition, (ii) their general health and (iii) their social background, eg. age, occupation etc. Given these facts, there were three categories into which they could place the patient: (i) within scope of practice but not legitimate use of time and skill (ii) within scope and legitimate use of time and skill (iii) beyond scope of practice. A pilot study revealed that this concept was quite foreign to many chiropodists and the introductory sheet underwent several metamorphoses. It also revealed that people wanted to qualify their choice of category, so a 'comments' column was added.

Some of the patients were drawn from actual experience, whilst other were deliberately constructed to pose difficult choices. Some had foot conditions for which the treatment is taught on courses leading to registration, but the sufferer did not come within the NHS priority groups. Similarly there were patients included who were suitable for footcare assistants, in order to detect how many registered chiropodists would refer down to these people. One patient was also included with a condition which a chiropodist ought to be able to diagnose but not to treat.

Whilst there were a few straightforward cases to help the chiropodists get used to the mechanics of the questionnaire, most were devised so that the case did not slot easily into one of the three categories. This was to force the chiropodist to consider carefully all the details which were provided before making a decision. The comments column proved to be well used. The combined results of 14 decisions on each questionnaire served to give a picture of how the chiropodist viewed his professional scope, indicating the upper and lower boundaries. When analysed in conjunction with the information regarding level and time of training and of their current employment, it would be possible to examine the influences which these factors have.

The sample

By definition, all state registered chiropodists must appear on the annually compiled Chiropodists Register. Details included in the register are names and addresses for each registrant, their registration number plus relevant qualifications. This list is alphabetical and a sample was taken on the basis of every tenth name, giving a list of 481 chiropodists. A total of 221 were returned completed, a response of 45.9%.

For the non-registered, obtaining a sample frame was less easy. There is no equivalent of the State Register. Non-registered chiropodists may or may not belong to one of the multiplicity of associations which open membership to them, but none of these organisations publish lists. The Institute of Chiropodists, which includes both registered and non-registered members, was prepared to help. While not giving us access to their membership list, the Institute provided names and addresses for 100 of its non-registered members. They were all sent questionnaires. The response rate was 42%.

Thus, there were, to begin with, two groups, registered and non-registered chiropodists. But from the information about them, lists of those working in the NHS and those in private practice were compiled. The registered chiropodists could also be grouped according to the year in which they commenced practice, which usually corresponds to when they completed training.

The decisions of over 250 chiropodists on 14 patients apiece naturally produced a great deal of interesting but very detailed information. For presentation in this book the results have been summarised and simplified. For each chiropodist, the 14 answers were divided into the three groups, sub-chiropody, chiropody, and supra-chiropody. Then the answers of all the registered chiropodists were added up. This shows their collective judgement on the percentages of the patients beyond, within and beneath their scope of practice. Thus as a group, registered chiropodists felt 17.5% of the patients fell in the supra-chiropodial class, and another 22% in the sub-chiropodial class. These were, in essence, the upper and lower limits of chiropody. In between fell the remaining 60.5% of patients whom they considered within their scope of practice. A similar calculation was carried out for the non-registered chiropodists and compared with the other results, to see whether they drew the boundaries of chiropody higher or lower than the registered. The same calculations and comparisons were done for public and private sector chiropodists, and for registrants trained in different periods. The differences between the groups are described in the text and set out graphically in Tables 31 to 33.

There are indeed considerable differences among chiropodists in the way they conceive chiropody. Broadly, these variations are in the direction which logic would suggest: registered, recently trained, and NHS chiropodists are more likely to accept patients with complex conditions and more likely to refuse patients with simple conditions.

Table 31: Position of 'chiropody' as defined by registered and non-registered chiropodists.

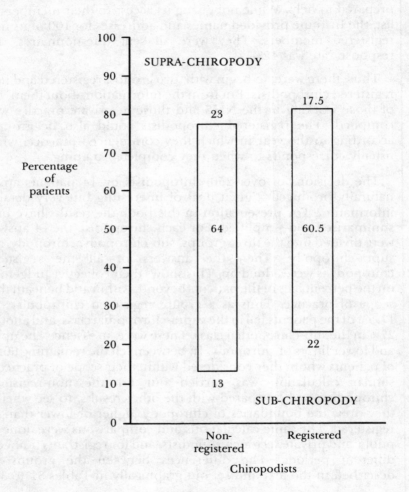

Registered *v.* non-registered

The most notable difference here is that the non-registered would accept patients with conditions lower down the footcare spectrum than the registered. They would decline to treat only 13% on grounds that they would involve an inappropriate use of their time and skills.

This willingness to undertake relatively low-skilled work may be explained, at least in part, by the fact that the non-registered work mostly in private practice, dependent on fees paid by patients for their livelihood. They literally cannot afford to turn people away, even if they feel that their skills are being underused.

From the graph it is also shown that the non-registered exclude more patients with conditions at the top end of the footcare spectrum. They would exclude 23% as beyond their scope, which has the effect of placing their upper boundary on the footcare spectrum at a lower level than given by registered chiropodists.

This may be due to the fact that, as their level of training is not so advanced as the level required for State Registration, some techniques are denied them and thus their scope may be restricted.

The registered are willing to take on more complex cases. They excluded only 17.5% of the test patients. Their sophistication was demonstrated in another way – their use of a 'comments' column provided on the questionnaire. Of their total decisions 22% were qualified or explained.

Only 8% of the responses from the non-registered were qualified in any way. It would thus seem that the registered view treatment decisions in a more complex and subtle way. An illustration of this was the emphasis put on seeking medical back-up or advice. Of the registered, 11% of their responses specified this action, as opposed to only 3% of the non-registered. This probably reflects the fact that whilst the registered are willing to treat more complex cases, they are also more inclined to consult others who are supervising the patient's other medical treatment. It is probably true in chiropody, as in other fields, that the more one is trained to do advanced techniques of any sort the more aware one ought to be of the factors which might complicate the procedure. Injecting local analgesics is a good example. The technique itself is relatively simple but it is vital to know details of such things as other drugs which may interact and cause collapse, the maximum safe dosage which may be given, how to deal with fainting or worse, etc. Many patients do not know the names of their drugs even if they know for what condition they are taken. Reference to the medical practitioner to gain or check information may frequently be necessary. This is also true when treating complicated cases such as are seen in many outpatient clinics in hospitals, where drug therapy may play an important part in the foot condition.

The differences are thus apparent, with the registered accepting more complex patients whilst rejecting more simple cases than their non-registered colleagues. The effect of these two factors is to give the registered a higher scope of practice, when drawn on the footcare spectrum.

When chiropodists commenced practice

The sample of registered chiropodists covers a long period of practice commencement: 1932 to 1980, a range of 49 years. This might be expected to produce variations in opinion, since those beginning in the 1980s have had a very different training from those who started practice almost half a century earlier. In order to see if, and how, this change influenced attitudes, groups within the sample were looked at using the date of commencement of practice as the basis for grouping.

The general picture produced is that the later-trained have a higher view of their scope of practice than the earlier groups. However, the earliest group of registered still have a higher view than the non-registered. This is consistent with the idea that training results in a different conception of chiropody.

Both boundaries show a straight line increase, with one exception in each case. The lower boundary, between sub-chiropody and chiropody, shows a slow but steady rise, right up to the last group. This may be because it takes experience and confidence to delegate tasks or refuse to carry out sub-chiropodial tasks for patients able to help themselves. The variation may thus be due to inexperience, or to the fact that the political issue of footcare assistants and closure of the profession has been aired more fully in the last few years. The one variation in the smooth increase of the upper boundary, the 1963/1967 group, is less easy to explain.

The training which chiropodists receive, as indicated by the date on which people commenced practice, does therefore have an effect on their views. At the lower end of the scale there appears to be a steady but progressive rise in the point at which registered chiropodists consider sub-chiropody to end, indicating a steady rise in expectations. At the upper end, there is a corresponding rise in where chiropodists view the limit of their scope of practice, reflecting the advances which an increasing understanding of foot function and pathology brings.

Table 32: Position of 'chiropody' as defined by registrants over last 22 years

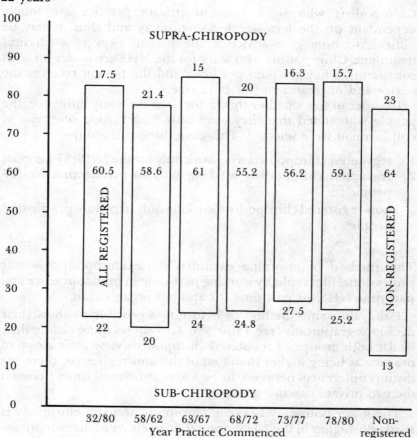

It would seem then that chiropodists are becoming more inclined to refuse low-skill work, or, for a few in the NHS, to delegate it. They also seem to be becoming more confident of their ability to treat more complex cases. The rise in the boundaries, however, both at the bottom and top ends, is quite small, These changes are happening, but very slowly.

Public sector *v.* private sector

Chiropodists who work only in private practice are totally dependant on the fees which patients pay and thus it may be difficult to only give advice if the patient expects a physical treatment. Chiropodists who work for the NHS are under no such constraints. They are paid per hour and the patient receives the advice and/or treatment free of charge.

In order to test whether this factor does have any influence, the people who stated that they were only undertaking one type of employment were selected. This gave three sub groups:

1.   registered chiropodists who work only for the NHS (87 people);
2.   registered chiropodists working only in private practice (27 people);
3.   non-registered chiropodists working only in private practice (37 people).

This method of grouping excluded those chiropodists whose professional life is split by working part-time in private practice and part-time NHS, or part-time for another organisation.

Using the same method as before it is possible to show their decisions graphically (see Table 33). This shows quite clearly that, whilst both groups of registered chiropodists view their scope of practice as being higher than that of the non-registered, there are distinct differences between the two, and some similarities between the two private practice groups.

The lower boundary between chiropody and sub-chiropody is markedly higher in the NHS group than in either of the two private practice groups. This reflects the fact that, in NHS employment, demands for pedicures can be refused without loss of income. In addition, refusal of a patient simply means that someone from a

Table 33: Position of 'chiropody' as determined by type of employment

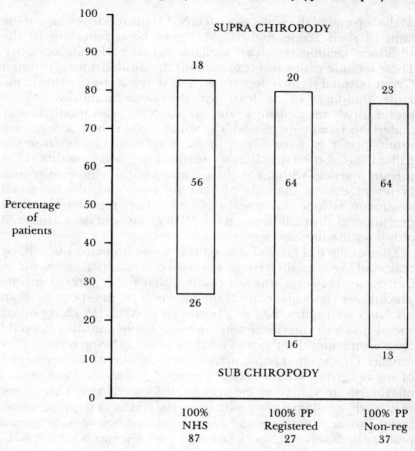

waiting list can be taken on for treatment, in private practice refusal may mean an empty appointment slot. There is also the fact that some NHS chiropodists may have footcare assistants to whom they can refer patients whose needs are for nail cutting only. The registered private practitioners are far closer to their non-registered colleagues, possible reflecting the dependence on fees, although they still draw the boundary higher up the scale.

Limit of their scope

At the top end of the scale, again it is NHS chiropodists who put the limit of their scope highest. This may be a reflection of the additional facilities which are available to many NHS chiropodists. These include easier access to patients' medical histories, through GPs or hospital records departments, as they may be working in the same building, or at least for the same authority. Where professional relationships are good, NHS chiropodists may undertake treatments for which, whilst within their scope, they would prefer to have advice or back-up available, because the patient has some complicating medical or social condition. In private practice, without such reassurance, the chiropodist may prefer to err on the side of caution, even though the actual treatment is one he uses regularly. The registered private practitioners thus fall between the NHS group and non-registered group on the footcare spectrum.

The results this far had proved that those influences which, by reason of logic, might have an effect on chiropodists' views, did in fact do so. However this last finding, that the registered private practitioner views his scope as slightly lower on the spectrum than his NHS colleagues, had not been predicted. NHS chiropodists spend much of their time with elderly people and thus it would have been logical for them to see their scope as being restricted by this fact. On the other hand, private practice, where patients may be of any age group with no 'priority groups', has always been seen as offering more variety in the chiropodist's workload. This is one reason why so many chiropodists view the NHS as a stepping stone, gaining some experience and a steady income before starting up a practice themselves. Others, of course, work sessions for the NHS as a means of providing a regular income as a supplement to the fees paid in their practice. For many, one of the attractions of private practice is the fact of being independent, another is the greater financial rewards which can be gained.

However, this research would appear to demonstrate that the variety in private practice is at the low skill end of the footcare spectrum, rather than at the higher end. The NHS thus actually has more to offer the chiropodist in terms of clinical advance than does private practice. If this is true, then the manpower crisis may be eased by the attraction of a bigger proportion of registered chiropodists into the NHS. However, unless the remuneration is made to compensate the loss of the other advantages of private practice, this will not happen, and even this would not solve the manpower crisis.

Narrower but higher scope of practice

Another interesting point from this division is the depth of the band designated 'chiropody' by each group, that is the distance between the lower and upper boundaries on the footcare spectrum. Both private practice groups have the same depth of band or range: 64% of patients included in 'chiropody'. The registered group view their range as occuring slightly higher on the spectrum. The NHS group, again viewing their scope as finishing further up the scale, also give a narrower band as being 'chiropody' – only 56%. This effectively means that they view themselves as having a narrower but higher scope of practice, perhaps a reflection of the fact that they are the experts on feet within the NHS, and therefore wish to delegate the simple tasks in order to become more widely recognised as such. Within other NHS professions this use of less highly trained staff is commonly found, and thus is a natural progression for chiropody.

Policy conclusions

The disinclination of NHS chiropodists to undertake low skill work has already created the space for a new sub-chiropodial role of footcare assistant. The rising lower boundary of chiropody among the more recently trained suggests that space will expand in future. This raising of standards leaves a range of skills which could be undertaken by less extensively trained people.

We can also see in the results of this study the basis for opposition to footcare assistants within the profession. It would appear that private practitioners still do undertake a substantial number of lower skill tasks, partly because there is a demand for such services, partly because they depend on patients' fees for their livelihood.

Even registered chiropodists in private practice carry out more low skill work than their counterparts in the NHS. But many of these people combine private practice with sessional work for the NHS. They may be the ones who have effectively resisted the introduction of footcare assistants. The fear of competition in the private sector appears to be having a potent spill-over effect on chiropody in the public sector. This is yet more evidence for the need to break the present stalemate.

Finally, we can see in these figures why other health professionals are uncertain about chiropody. Chiropodists have varied opinions themselves. We can also see why other potential referrers underestimate chiropodists' skills. Many chiropodists still do accept patients whose needs involve only low skill work. Clarifying the conception of chiropody and increasing the range of referrals will not be a simple task.

Part V

Reforming Footcare: Policy and Practice

22 Introduction

At the end of each of the earlier chapters, policy changes have been suggested for all the groups which participate in footcare and which, therefore, will be involved in bringing about improvement. In this conclusion, all these scattered recommendations are brought together into one summary statement of possible reforms to policy and practice in footcare.

Each group involved in footcare is considered in turn. Each section is designed to be self-contained, but since the footcare world is complex, with overlapping needs and roles, any change in one area will have multiple and far-reaching effects, on both the providers and users of services. Some repetition is therefore inevitable.

Chiropody services are dealt with first for two reasons. First, this study originated with a chiropodist and it is felt that chiropodists have to put their own house in order first, and secondly, if the other changes are to occur, chiropodists have to create the extra capacity to provide more treatments to a wider range of patients, which necessitates a change in their philosophy. To achieve these changes will not be easy, but can it be demonstrated that some at least are possible in the short term?

23 Chiropodists: change underway

The changes necessary in chiropody fall naturally into two categories: local and national. The policy changes which have been agreed in the district where the field work took place indicate that there is scope for changes at the local level. These will be described first, followed by a discussion of the policy issues which require action from chiropodists and others at higher than service delivery level.

Local policy issues

One of the most important findings of this research was the proportion of people already receiving or waiting for chiropody treatment who did not need 'chiropody' at all but foot hygiene— nail cutting. Many of the unmet needs in the community were also for this less skilled, sub-chiropodial type of service. The estimates of the proportion of current patients who needed only sub-chiropodial treatments from chiropodists ranged from a minimum of 10% to a maximum of 58%. Before the research had begun a post for an FCA had been created, but not filled. Since documenting the true extent of need for foot hygiene, the chiropody service has gone on to employ three FCAs. The nail cutting service is thus operating in a variety of sites, wherever it is possible to have the supervising chiropodist and FCA working together.

As repeatedly indicated during this report, the use of FCAs is a politically contentious issue. Some difficulty might have been anticipated in introducing so many assistants into the existing service. On the contrary, a significant raising of the morale of chiropodists has occurred. They no longer have to give low skill treatments except where medical complications bring nail cutting into a high skill task; nor to answer the telephone or enquiries; and having an assistant also raises their status in the eyes of patients and other professional staff.

The investigation of the waiting list revealed two kinds of inadequacy: in the referral procedure itself and in the way in which the forms were dealt with after receipt at chiropody headquarters. Two different types of referral forms, both incomplete, were in use for (i) professionals and (ii) potential patients. This carried the risk of giving more emphasis to 'professional' forms regardless of the information given. The professional form requested much medical information but had no question about the foot condition for which the referral was being made. The self referral form asked why chiropody was wanted but sought little medical information. Both medical and foot condition have a bearing on the urgency of need. On arrival at the chiropody office the forms were scanned for any indication of urgency and, where none was detected, filed chronologically on the waiting list. Urgent referrals were given appointments, but that depended on the referrer volunteering additional information on the form.

New referral form

In response to these defects, a new referral form has been designed, using the best from each of the old forms; and assessment clinics for all new patients have been introduced. The new form is designed to give an indication of urgency so that the most urgent patients are given an immediate assessment. Non-urgent cases, as judged from the form, are given assessment appointments within a month of application. The referral form has also been designed to allow the applicant, or assessing chiropodist, to provide all the necessary information for the new computerised appointment system being introduced.

One of the most distressing discoveries from the waiting list study was the fact that it contained people who needed treatment immediately. With the appointment system blocked, and a waiting time of a year, there was no way for them to gain immediate access to treatment.

The assessment appointment which all new applicants receive is an extension of the waiting list study. The medical history, capacity for self help, and footwear styles and attitudes are explored and a chiropodial examination carried out. Any necessary advice is given and the patient either given an appointment or returned to the waiting list until a vacancy occurs. If an appointment for treatment is given this may be for foot hygiene from an FCA or for intensive chiropody. In this way, neither patients needing urgent treatment nor only foot hygiene are returned to the waiting list. All the chiropodists have been taught a standard assessment procedure to ensure parity across the district.

One of the major problems is that NHS chiropody services are frequently organised so that they predominantly give routine maintenance treatments rather than making intensive attempts to cure and discharge the patient. This is a major contribution to the blockage of the service and to the 'manpower shortage'. The research revealed that there was a substantial scope for intensive curative treatments, which would result in a reduction in the district's workload.

This system, whilst designed principally with new patients in mind, in order to bring them to optimum foot health in the minimum number of appointments, has also proved useful for some existing patients. Not all existing patients can have much further improvement made in their feet, either for clinical reasons or because they are unwilling to change their shoe styles, but some are only too happy to co-operate in an intensive effort to improve their conditions.

In order to allow such intensive treatments to take place, a reorganisation of the chiropodists' schedules has occurred. Each now has sessions during the week in which he or she is free to book patients for whatever time-span they require, rather than the standard system of all patients being booked for identical periods of time.

This, along with the introduction of FCAs, is acting to unblock the appointment system. The gains from intensive treatment sessions are not only a greater ability to give patients the type of service they need, but, just as importantly, the chiropodists have increased job satisfaction. They have more variety in their work, and 'the system' is no longer preventing them from using all their persuasive and curative skills to bring patients to optimum foot health.

Whilst the intensive approach does create vacancies for new patients, it does not affect the numerical size of the waiting list. If anything, the list is larger now than ever. This is due to the fact that people do not apply for chiropody if they can see no hope of ever receiving treatment. However, if the waiting list is seen to move, with people coming off the list and onto the service, people again start to apply.

Whilst the introduction of assessment clinics will ensure that those whose needs are 'urgent' at the time of referral/application are given appointments, it will not prevent people's condition deteriorating whilst on the 'assessed waiting list'. To deal with this problem, an emergency clinic has been set up. Anyone, on the waiting list, currently receiving treatment or not in contact with the service at all, may attend.

The procedures for running this clinic have been carefully thought out so that it remains a facility for treating emergencies and does not become a means for people with minor foot problems to jump the waiting list queue. Anyone with a foot condition which they consider urgent may attend the Central Chiropody Clinic without an appointment on any weekday morning.

Only the condition causing pain is treated and patients cannot be seen as an emergency again within four weeks. Where the chiropodist wishes to see them sooner they are given an appointment for an appropriate date. If people are current chiropody patients, their treatment is investigated to see if there is any reason why they should have developed an 'emergency'. If they are on the waiting list they may be returned to it, or given an appointment if that is more appropriate. People who are not on the list are, if it is thought in their interest, encouraged to apply. Those presenting with non-urgent conditions are turned away with the appropriate advice as to what they should do about their problem.

This emegency facility has proved extremely popular and, even with these restrictions, is oversubscribed. It is not a particularly easy clinic for the staff, as people often do no want to accept the emergency rules, but it is obviously fulfilling a real need. It does relieve pressure on the clerical staff, who do at least now have somewhere to send people who have not yet received routine appointments.

Advice has appeared as a 'need' in many places throughout this text. One policy change planned but not yet in action is an advisory clinic. This will not give treatment of any sort but will exist to give advice on self care of the feet, or on care of children's or old people's feet and on footwear. Many people are unaware of even the rudiments of how to purchase suitable shoes. Commercially available shoes will be inadequate for some people, but for many people simple guidelines would be of great assistance. It is envisaged that the advisory service could see many of the working people who seek treatment but who are at present receiving nothing in terms of footcare from the NHS unless they have an acute condition, such as an ingrown nail or an injury. The advisory service would of course refer people with conditions requiring treatment to the appropriate agency.

Self care course

Again, on the theme of helping people to help themselves, or others, two more schemes have been devised. The first is an experimental self care course being run in conjunction with a local health group, set up for people on a large housing estate. The idea was to provide the participants with the knowledge to care for their own feet as far as is safe and particularly to help them choose and wear suitable shoes. The health workers who run the scheme helped to prepare broadsheets and consultation took place with a representative of the intended target group so that their point of view was known. It was hoped that the health workers would also act as 'shopping' aides, helping the less mobile to the shops to choose shoes. Unfortunately, this first attempt proved to be a lesson in how not to do it. Despite the production of broadsheets inviting people to attend, the turnout was poor and, as the only space available was a large hall, the setting was far from ideal. The fact that the speaker was a chiropodist also proved to be disadvantageous, as the people saw it as an opportunity to make enquiries about why they were not getting any (or enough) treatment from the NHS, rather than tackling the subject of self help. Future sessions have been planned, but in a rather different format in an attempt to avoid such problems.

The second scheme, aimed at prevention or early detection of foot problems is a workshop for school nurses. School nurses have much to offer in terms of foot health if they are given more knowledge. Closer co-operation will, it is hoped, mean that more children will be referred for both advice and treatment. If successful, it may be practical to set up workshops for other care groups such as health visitors, district nurses, staff of community old people's homes, community health workers and the bathing attendants who visit old people in their own homes to help them with bathing.

All the changes involve the chiropodists in extra work. However, the effect has been to raise morale, rather than depress it. Giving the chiropodists an increased variety in their work has been good for them as it stretches their abilities, making them use all their skills. There will always be the routine work but this is viewed much more positively when it does not take up their whole professional lives.

One of the most common outcomes of all social research is the recommendation of more research. That conclusion is perhaps more justified here than in most studies. It has many times been stressed that this research was undertaken with very limited resources – one person working for one year with virtually no funds. The result was compromises in the choice of research methods. In each of the chapters describing the substudies, the ideal way to investigate the problem was repeatedly pointed out, along with actual methods used.

In consequence, this has not been as methodologically correct a study as could and should be done. But nevertheless the results, in terms of discovering unmet needs and the inefficiencies in the provision of footcare, are dramatic. So much so, that the district has pressed on with the reforms of the service just described. But the data base on which these conclusions and changes have been grounded is not as solid as it could be.

Therefore, the most important form of 'further research' which should be undertaken is a comprehensive and methodologically correct replication of the need and current provision studies.

New initiatives in provision

Two research projects have already been started. One is a further study of elderly people, who featured so largely in this research. The new study will explore in depth alternative methods of providing footcare treatments to elderly people, with the emphasis on the foot hygiene end of the footcare spectrum. The object is to enable as many elderly people as possible to enjoy foot comfort without becoming dependant on chiropody treatment as there will never be enough chiropodists to treat everyone. Maintenance of mobility and independence are of course important to both the individual and to the State. A variety of experimental models are proposed and will be tested over a two year period.

The other study, of diabetics, has been proposed by a contact made during this research. The study is examining the clinical effects of treatment regimes for diabetics, and the chiropodists are involved in the monitoring and treatment of foot conditions. Both projects have the advantage of giving direct treatment to patients with existing needs and are thus of practical benefit as well as making academic advance. The time to do such things is coming from the increased efficiency within the existing service.

Table 34: Summary of changes in research district

1	Referral forms	The existing two have been redesigned into one new one
2	Waiting list	Compilation procedures revised
3	Assessment clinics	For all applicants
4	Foot hygiene service	For simple nail cutting
5	Treatment plans	For all patients
6	Positive attitudes	Motivation of chiropodists
7	Intensive clinics	Allows intensive treatment to bring feet to optimum condition
8	Emergency clinic	For urgent conditions
9	Training workshops	For other health professionals
10	Self care courses	For community health groups
11	Educational material	New leaflets, broadsheets
12	Advisory clinic	On footwear and self help
13	Diabetic research	To improve preventive care
14	Research project on elderly people	To explore alternative service delivery models

There have therefore been many changes within this particular chiropody service. Some have been a success, others less so. The purpose of the description of these changes, however, is not to propose a model for copying. Some other health districts already have some of the services described, and not all changes will be necessary or, indeed, possible elsewhere. The aim, rather, is to demonstrate that changes are actually possible that do not cost much in financial terms.

National policy issues

A number of national policy issues have been mentioned throughout this book which appertain to chiropodists. The major ones are: training, research, sub-chiropodial manpower, and closure of the profession.

1. Training

The recognised training is primarily undertaken in the schools of chiropody in the United Kingdom, using the examinations set by the Society of Chiropodists. This training and the qualification gained after passing the examinations are approved by the Chiropodists Board and allow entry onto the state register. State registration is a condition of employment within the NHS (see page 24) and thus if the number of NHS chiropodists is to rise, expansion of the number of training places needs to continue, both by increasing the intake at existing schools and by opening new ones. The Society of Chiropodists should encourage more practitioners to become teachers, at present in short supply. It should also be actively campaigning for mandatory grants for students who wish to take its training course and examinations.

If some form of closure comes about, the Society would also, presumably, become involved in the training of sub-chiropodial manpower. There would have to be regulation of the syllabus taught, and many Society members would be involved in that training.

2. Research

One of the other problems which besets chiropody is the comparative lack of research, both social and clinical. As has been stressed, the research described in this book was done with limited resources and this imposed limitations on both the methods of investigation and on the size of the total project.

There are many other areas in chiropody where social policy research could add greatly to our knowledge, for example by investigating uptake, the value of providing transport as opposed to domiciliary visits and the provision of surgical footwear. The latter is a source of much frustration to patients and chiropodists alike.

Equally, clinical research in chiropody is still in its infancy. A lot of work is being done in the United States, and some work on foot function is now being started in this country. Technological changes, especially computers, are making much more possible than in the past. However, many of the problems of the skin are still poorly understood, as is the case in medicine, and this could be a valuable area for investigation. In some cases, whilst treatment is known to be safe and effective, the reason why this should be so is unclear.

Of course, with the present manpower shortage it is not being suggested that chiropodists all become researchers in the more esoteric branches of their work, but there is great scope for epidemiological studies in their daily work.

3. Sub-chiropodial manpower and closure of the profession

These two issues are considered together, as the authors feel that they are intimately connected. It has been shown that there is a vast need for expanding the footcare provision available in a controlled and systematic way.

The DHSS did attempt to introduce the grade of Footcare Assistant in 1977, against resistance from the Society of Chiropodists. The Society wanted to resolve the issue of closure of the profession first. In practice, the chiropodists working in the NHS effectively blocked the usage of such personnel, and their duties are still restricted to the cutting of normal nails. The chiropodists resisted because of concern about creating a pool of poorly trained, inadequately regulated people who could set up in practice as 'chiropodists'.

The debate about closure continued, and the last attempt at an agreement on closure was the consultative document entitled 'Proposals for statutory protection of professional titles under the Professionals Supplementary to Medicine Act, 1960 and closure of the speech therapy profession'. After consultations with the various professions, including chiropody, it was decided that 'it would not be right to put forward proposals during the lifetime of this Parliament for amending legislation either for functional closure or for indicative closure of these professions'. The reason given was that 'Among the professions concerned there was no clear consensus nor common ground'. However, the letter to Regional Administrators in the NHS went on to say that the Government was 'anxious to make progress on this issue'. This is a recognition that the issue will not go away, and that the current stalemate must be broken. The pressures of work and the level of unmet need will continue to rise, as will the cost, in both humanitarian and financial terms, of inefficient use of existing resources.

Without taking any position on the ultimate resolution of this issue, it is clear that both sides, chiropodists and the DHSS, must come to some agreement. Once this has happened, the number of FCAs would rise, as they would no longer be seen as potential competitors, and with suitable training would have expanded duties analagous perhaps to those of a dental hygienist, especially where the patient really only wants or needs routine treatment akin to pedicure. This, in turn, would release chiropodists for more highly skilled work.

From both the description of the national issues, and the actual changes made in the research district, it will be seen that there are many areas of policy change in which chiropodists can be instrumental, both individually and collectively.

24 The shoe trade: selling us short

The shoe trade, both in the shoes it manufactures, and in the way it sells them, has a great influence on the nation's foot health. Shoes are not the only cause of foot problems, but they are implicated.

Manufacturers

Some manufacturers already spend a good deal of time, money and effort making shoes which come in width fittings and half sizes. However, they are few in number, and their products are inevitably in the higher price range. This is due, at least in part, to the extra investment required to make any given style in several width fittings, as well as in more sizes. With fashion changing from season to season, there is also a risk that not all these shoes will be sold which would represent a trade loss.

In children's ranges, only a few makes come in a full range of width fittings and half sizes, despite the fact that only 50% of children can be fitted in an average width shoe. Ideally, all children should have properly fitted shoes changed regularly as their feet grow. But as these shoes are often rather expensive, many parents, unable to afford to replace them as often as necessary, try to make them last longer, until gradually they become too short and tight for the children's feet (see Table 28). There is a good case for cheaper, width fitted shoes which have built-in obsolescence.

Elderly people also have problems in buying suitable shoes. For many, even the widest standard fittings found in shops are inadequate, and they are thus forced to wear badly fitting footwear. Many wear slippers indoors all day, and few slippers on the market have a fastening.

A revolution in slipper design is needed, so that there is an alternative to the present restricted choice. It is not impossible to produce a soft shoe, with a fastening, which resembles a slipper, but which has the advantage of being constructed like a properly fitting shoe. Fastenings do not have to be difficult. 'Touch and close' materials are quite effective, as are zip fasteners. Both of these can be used by people who need a dressing stick or other aid to dress themselves. Elderly people, whilst not the wealthiest consumers when considered individually, do represent a rapidly growing market force. They should be taken seriously. There could be a large commercial opportunity for firms which design attractive footwear for elderly people and which gain a reputation for value-for-money. The organisations which promote the welfare of elderly people could take the initiative in pointing out this specialist market to manufacturers, recommending appropriate design and organising purchase to make it worthwhile.

Influence of fashion

The subject of fashion has been raised several times. The influence of fashion is large, and will always operate in the footwear market. However, at present, it is very difficult for many women to purchase shoes which both fit and are pleasing to the eye. Whilst the problem can, to some extent, be avoided by wearing different shoes for work and dress wear, it would be much more beneficial if fashion and foot health could work together, rather than in opposite directions. Since it is impossible to change the factors affecting foot health, it is the factors which operate in fashion that must be changed. The recent trend in increased participation in sports has brought some fashionable lace-ups into the shops, but these are really only for wear with leisure clothes and not with more formal dress. The dualism in shoe design between the 'sensible' and the 'fashionable', must be eliminated. Manufacturers should make practical shoes that look good and trendy shoes that fit.

On the retail side, the shoe shops and their assistants are potentially the largest core of health educators in the field. Some already promote foot health but there is much to be gained by promoting the idea of the right shoe for the job. For the trade, it is better to sell two pairs of shoes, rather than one. It could also be beneficial for foot health if people wear one shoe for work and a more fashionable one for leisure time. This is not an appropriate message for those with feet still growing, as 'best' shoes will be outgrown before they are out-worn, but may be acceptable for adults whose feet change more slowly.

Trained assistants

An increased number of trained assistants in shops could also help, encouraging and enabling people to have their feet measured at every purchase. The best policy would be not to sell shoes unless they were fitted, but this is impractical in the real world. Self service in shoe shops and large stores is an increasing trend, which is not especially desirable from the foot health perspective, particularly where children's shoes are concerned. Even these shops could play a part, however, by having assistants who were trained to at least a basic standard, and by providing guidance to customers on shoe fitting in the form of do-it-yourself measuring gauges, wall charts, etc.

Mail order is another growing trend. The standard of instructions given for ordering varies tremendously. Simply giving the sizes available is little help, as the way in which different styles fit affects the size required. For some elderly and handicapped people, especially those with no available transport to take them to a shop with a fitting service, mail order may be the only solution. So long as the ordering instructions are as clear as possible, including guidance, for example on the need for shoes to be longer than the foot (a point many people overlook), mail order may not be too undesirable. For children, mail order is not a good idea as their feet need to be measured regularly. The temptation with mail order is that once the goods have arrived, they are accepted even if they are not quite what is needed.

Another policy which could be adopted is the labelling of shoes with the type of wear for which they are designed, eg. occasional, wet weather, etc. Some companies already do this, and it would not only help by educating consumers to think of 'shoes for the occasion' but also reduce the complaints about quality from customers who had actually bought a shoe for the wrong type of wear.

In sum, the shoe trade has a contribution to make to foot health at every stage of its activities.

25 Voluntary organisations:
unorganised potential

Various voluntary organisations are already involved in providing footcare services. However, their potential contribution has not been fully developed and, since the schemes already running are not co-ordinated on a large scale, the voluntary sector may be seen as disorganised.

Voluntary organisations could make substantial contributions to the footcare services in six distinct areas: nail cutting, accommodation, education, transport, shopping aids and finance.

Different types of nail cutting services were described earlier (see page 131), and these met with different responses from state registered chiropodists. Again, as with FCAs, volunteers may set themselves up in practice as chiropodists, so that such schemes are not always welcome. Voluntary organisations have to recognise the existence of this problem, and adopt a strategy which avoids conflict whilst continuing to provide a service to those they seek to help. As a matter of policy they should seek the co-operation of the local District Chiropody Service, which may be willing to provide supervision, and guidelines on the types of people to whom such nail cutting services should not be offered. Where such joint organisation and supervision exist, the voluntary organisations may find their services more readily accepted. The five remaining areas of potential help are less controversial.

In the past, accommodation has frequently been provided by voluntary organisations in village or church halls in areas where there was little statutory building. With the changes in chiropody training and the increasing sophistication of the equipment used by chiropodists, accommodation in such halls may no longer be acceptable. However, many voluntary organisations now have new buildings which may incorporate a multi-purpose medical room, or indeed, a chiropody surgery. If voluntary organisations wish to continue their fine record of providing space for a chiropodist to work, they must recognise the changing standards which are increasingly expected, and found, by chiropodists within the National Health Service.

Voluntary clerical help and reception staff are often welcomed although sensitivity must be exercised, however, if conflict with the trade unions is to be avoided.

Appropriately trained volunteers could undertake a broad educational role, including giving talks to groups on the subjects of foot health, self help, footwear and its importance, and on how and when to seek professional advice. The format of these talks could vary from small group sessions, with shoe fitting demonstrations, to larger lectures to women's meetings, pensioners' groups, etc. Volunteers could also produce, with appropriate professional advice, broadsheets, leaflets, posters and other educational material fort distribution to interested parties. Short presentations on tape or video could also be prepared.

One problem which faces many chiropodists who give talks is that people always want a professional opinion on their individual case, which rather defeats the purpose of the session. The other common problem is that the chiropodist is seen as representing 'authority' and thus becomes a target for all the dissatisfaction about the inadequate number of appointments available. Using a volunteer who could not become involved in this way would avoid this problem.

Many voluntary groups provide or organise transport in a variety of ways, eg. private cars, mini-buses, etc., for trips to many events, from hospital appointments to outings. Schemes to take people, otherwise housebound, to NHS chiropody clinics already exist. Such schemes reduce the need for domiciliary (home) visits which are both time consuming and costly.

The fifth area in which voluntary organisations could provide a service is by organising 'shopping aides' (or volunteers) who would help handicapped or elderly people who are unsteady on their feet or who cannot use public transport without help, to purchase suitable shoes. A volunteer with the time to visit local shops and identify those with shoe fitters and/or suitable ranges of shoes would be invaluable to those for whom shopping is difficult. The shopping aide could also talk to shop managers and thus attempt to improve the services available.

If no shoe fitter were available, a simple training of volunteers in the rudiments of shoe fitting would also reduce the number of purchases which were totally unsuitable, which pensioners at least can ill afford. Control would obviously have to be exercised to prevent shopping aides from becoming unofficial sales representatives of any particular retailer or manufacturer.

The final area of activity for voluntary organisations is in providing funds for research work into the needs of their particular interest groups and in alternative ways to provide for those needs.

In this outline of possible areas of action for voluntary organisations, opportunities have been described which exist for the unorganised potential to become auxilliary helpers in the footcare world without coming into conflict with the statutory services.

26 Social services departments: enabling footcare

The role of social services departments in footcare is a varied one, with several types of staff and service involved.

1. Social workers

One function of a social worker is to visit people, investigate their needs, and arrange for these needs to be met wherever possible. Whilst it is impossible for all social workers to know everything, they should know, or be able to find out, where and how other statutory services are provided.

In the study of handicapped people, it was found that many of the subjects, whilst recognising a need for footcare, did not think it worth applying to the local chiropody service because they thought that they would not get it. It was not clear why they held this opinion, but it is wrong, and both chiropodists and social workers have a duty to see that people are properly informed. This is especially true of the subjects studied, as many were both handicapped and elderly. Additionally, social workers have access to transport which can be utilised to take otherwise housebound people to clinics for treatment.

2. Day centres and residential homes

Many day centres for elderly and handicapped people of all ages are run by social services. In many cases the NHS chiropody service is unable (through lack of staff) or unwilling (due to lack of facilities) to run treatment sessions in day centres. However, chiropody assessment sessions could possibly be held in the centres, as the only facilities required are privacy, a desk, chairs and foot rest and wash hand basin.

In some health districts, the district chiropodist will arrange for staff to visit homes to give footcare treatments, either chiropody or nail cutting. In others, care staff are taught to cut normal nails, with a chiropodist screening all clients for suitability. Those needing more than simple nail cutting are then looked after by the chiropodist, the rest by the care staff. Staff can also help by giving advice to patients or their relatives regarding suitable shoes for wear both in the home and outside it. It may also be possible to arrange, with the help of the local chiropody service, for a shoe fitter to hold an occasional session for people wishing to buy shoes, but who find difficulty in doing so at a shop.

3. Advisers to the disabled

Social services departments also employ 'advisers to the disabled' – usually qualified occupational therapists who prefer to get out of hospitals and work in the community. These advisers may see clients at day centres or in their own homes. Of the large number of aids available to make daily life easier for handicapped people, some relate to footcare. Knowing about, and obtaining, these aids may allow a handicapped or elderly person to retain independence in everyday activities, even if cutting the nails is beyond their capability.

Advisers should also be aware that ranges of special footwear are available for both children and adults. The Disabled Living Foundation (see Appendix III) has two collections of specimen shoes and aids, one for children and one for adults, which may be hired. It also publishes books on the subject (see Appendix IV). Appointments can also be made for advisers and clients to visit the Foundation for advice.

None of the suggestions made for social services departments' participation in footcare are particularly difficult to achieve, nor do they involve much extra cost. It is important, however, that the co-operation of the local National Health Service is sought before embarking on certain of the suggestions, as success will depend on liaison between the two services.

27 Nurses: community outreach

This section is subdivided into various types of nursing staff, who have different roles in the promotion of foot health.

1. Hospital-based nurses

The basic nursing qualifications are gained by both theoretical and practical training in hospitals. The hospital nurses will be involved in the care of patients' feet, including general skin care, the prevention and treatment of pressure sores. They will also cut toenails for patients whose conditions do not bring such a procedure into the chiropodist's sphere. In many cases, chiropodists find that nursing staff, like many doctors, have a rather narrow view of a chiropodist's scope of practice, and so tend to refer only patients who require nail cutting. This is probably due to (i) a deficiency in the training of nurses, and (ii) a lack of initiative on the part of chiropodists to make good this deficiency, and their acquiescence in the role assigned to them through inappropriate referrals.

2. Community-based nurses

Three groups are relevant here: district nurses, health visitors, and school nurses.

(i) District nurses

Whilst little has been said in this book about district nurses, it is recognised that they play a large part in the care of people in the community, not least amongst elderly people. They visit their patients regularly, and carry out on their behalf a large number of treatments and services. One service which some perform is the cutting of normal nails, but this practice is not universal. Often, however, they help with washing the feet if the old people cannot cope for themselves. Although it is recognised that district nurses already carry a heavy work load, they might be able to include foot hygiene in the general care. For a chiropodist to make separate visits for such a simple task would seem to be a costly use of manpower. It may be argued that chiropodists frequently recognise potential dangers even in people who only require nail cutting, but it is presumptuous to believe that a properly trained nurse could not do the same. Practical training sessions for district nurses, during which they learn to cut nails easily, to recognise danger signs in the feet and to give basic footwear advice, would be neither costly nor difficult to arrange locally. They could also learn about the role of chiropodists and how to use the chiropody service wisely. Chiropodists, likewise, would learn more about district nursing.

(ii) Health visitors

Health visitors are usually associated with the care of the very young and families with young children. In some districts, however, health visitors now have a more expanded role as family visitors, which brings them into contact with all age groups. Other health visitors spend a much greater proportion of their time with elderly people. In all groups, but particularly the very young and old, the health visitor has a definite foot health role.

In small babies, the potential for damage to feet is very high. The pressure from tight blankets has been recognised as potentially harmful to the feet and should be avoided.

Hose, such as tights or the leggings of all-in-one garments, can also be harmful. Ingrown toe nails are seen in children not yet standing, possibly due to the pressure of the garment.

More importantly the toes may buckle due to the pressure caused by the attempted contraction of the fibres in the garment.

The health visitor can thus educate mothers on dangers and should advocate the purchase of leggings, tights or sleep suits which do not have integral stretch 'feet'. Health visitors are ideally placed to advise when the first shoe should be worn. They could also teach mothers the importance of fitting shoes properly, the danger of the child outgrowing the shoe and that this outgrowing causes damage without the child experiencing pain. Health visitors, knowing the circumstances of the families they visit, can give more sensitive advice on shoe purchase than chiropodists, who may not realise that a mother may not be able (for financial reasons) to take well meaning (and idealistic) advice on width fittings and leather uppers, and so be discouraged from trying to do the best she can afford. Health visitors also have a role in referring or introducing an anxious mother to the chiropody service, which caters for children free of charge.

Health visitors also come into contact with expectant mothers, who, it was found, tend to have foot problems connected with the pregnancy rather than directly with the feet. The research did however indicate a need for advice, and this could quite easily be given by the health visitor. She could advise on how to obtain chiropody treatment if it were needed, acting as a link between the maternity service and the chiropodist. Health visitors could also be taught screening, in the same way as school nurses.

In their role as visitors to elderly people, much of the above also applies. Advice on footwear would be a major input, with the health visitor having the advantage of greater insight into individual problems and circumstances. Many elderly people who are not totally housebound spend much of their time at home, and it has been shown that in the effect it has on the feet, indoor footwear is probably more important than outdoor. Discouragement of slipper wearing may be more effective on the grounds of safety than on foot health, and health visitors are able to observe danger areas in the home. They may also be able to advise on how best to cope with the problem of nail cutting and washing of the feet. These tasks are often much less simple for those with arthritis, who find it difficult to bend and balance.

Health visitors are, then, an existing resource with a potentially expanded role in the footcare world, provided they receive sufficient training in this area.

The importance of foot health would need to be brought to their attention, since it would add yet another responsibility to an already considerable load.

(iii) School nurses

School nurses have a key role to play in foot health care, particularly in prevention. Little preventive work is being done at present: chiropodists are in short supply and the shoe trade, which could have great influence by promoting good practice in shoe purchase, has largely abdicated its responsibility.

School nurses are already involved in foot health but their involvement at present is not as effective as it might be, simply because they have not received sufficient training. This is not intended as a criticism of the nurses themselves, rather of the training which they receive and of chiropodists who may have done little to encourage school nurses to become more involved. Most nurses included in the study actively welcomed the involvement, and the chance to learn more about the feet they were inspecting. At present, they appear to concentrate on the detection of skin lesions such as warts, athlete's foot and also ingrown toe nails, rather than on skeletal problems. More emphasis on detection of long term skeletal problems would be useful, and would not preclude continuing detection of skin lesions.

The school physical examination provides a clear example of how an existing resource is not used to best advantage. A screening system already exists, but it does not work as effectively as it could and should.

Any improvement in the effectiveness of the screening system would, however, have implications for the chiropody service. First, it would need to become involved in training, but more importantly, would need to create the capacity for treating the extra children referred. This, unlike training, would have continuous, long term effects on the chiropody service. At present, only 2.8% of clinical chiropody time is spent on school children. If the level of unmet need is as high as suggested by the present research, this proportion of time will have to rise.

The research showed, however, that there were not only problems with the feet, but also with footwear. Sadly, it was not possible to include hose in the research, although its importance is acknowledged. It became apparent that the school nurse did not see the children wearing their shoes, which were frequently carried or left outside the room. An inspection of the feet, shod as well as bare, would obviously lengthen the examination time, but would allow detection of poorly fitting or outgrown footwear. It will be remembered that inadequate footwear was noted in 71% of the children surveyed. The extra time taken would be more than repaid if it prevented the child from becoming one of the 88% of old people who have foot trouble. School nurses are already involved in communicating with parents, and could therefore include advice to parents, in the new, more effective screening role. They would thus become foot health educators, both to the child and to the parent.

In order to make these changes in procedure, closer links would be required between the chiropody and school nursing services. Training by chiropodists could be given on the job and at specially organised workshops and study days.

In all three branches of nursing discussed here, it is up to the chiropodists to take the initiative in providing motivation and practical training if district nurses, health visitors and school nurses are to fulfil the expanded roles suggested here. None of the reforms would be costly and, although all four services would be increasing their workload, the greater load would bring increased use of skills and, in consequence, increased job satisfaction.

28 Education authorities: multiple opportunities

Schools and education authorities could help to prevent foot problems in four major ways.

First, by having a policy on school footwear, but with important provisos. As shoes and socks are virtually the only clothes which can damage the wearer's health, it would be sensible to minimise this possibility by advocating straightforward, common sense rules, ie. that they should have a fastening across the instep, flat heels and no 'flip-flops' (on safety grounds). These rules would neither discriminate against the less well off, nor restrict parental choice too much. The fact that the school had any rules about footwear would at least bring to parents' notice the fact that it is important, but need not be inordinately expensive. If a simple guide to foot health and children's shoes accompanied the rules it would explain why the school felt it desirable to have such rules.

Secondly, foot health is a task for teachers, as the long term improvement in standards of foot health will only come about through education. Most schools teach health education but foot health can be introduced into other subjects, using projects built around footwear. Shoe styles are influenced by the wearer's geographical location and by the historical period in which he lives (or lived). The materials from which shoes are made are also a source of interest.

Teachers should be encouraged to design and develop teaching aids, using the local chiropody service to provide factual background information. Local celebrities or historic places could also be involved, making the teaching aid relevant and interesting.

Since the class teacher is usually the person who helps the school nurse during hygiene inspections, the teacher and nurse can co-operate to promote a foot health message. If 'Foot Health Week' (see page 200) becomes an annual event as it is in the United States, this week could become the focal point for such collaboration.

Schools also have a responsibility for policies regarding the wearing of shoes and socks for gymnastics and other indoor activities. These policies take into account safety and hygiene, but should also include some consideration of the effects of barefoot exercise on foot health. For the vast majority, this is beneficial, but there are exceptions, even when the environment is safe. Likewise, many schools have swimming lessons, either in their own pool or at a public one. Opinion is divided on whether children with *verrucae* should be allowed to go swimming or not, but the decision should at least be based on logic, unlike one school which ordered children with *verrucae* (warts) to change and stand alongside the pool but not to enter the water!

Finally, it is education authorities who allocate grants for further education. At present, grants for chiropody students are discretionary, not mandatory (like grants for degree courses). This means that some local education authorities may refuse a grant application from someone wishing to become a state registered chiropodist. Local education authorities should be made aware of the acute shortage of NHS chiropodists and persuaded to look favourably on applications for grants, whilst the Department of Education and Science should move to make grants mandatory.

29 Doctors: renegotiating boundaries

It is clear that, as a general policy, doctors should transfer more patients to the chiropody service. At present, expensive medical resources are used inefficiently in that both family and hospital doctors are dealing with many foot complaints which could be handled by others. The aim should be to increase the referral of those patients who are within the scope of practice of chiropodists. The way in which this improved matching of problems to personnel is achieved will vary with the different types of doctors. But three steps need to be undertaken with all doctors: education, negotiation and re-organisation.

Many doctors are, understandably, ignorant about chiropody. They are not aware of recent developments within the profession, if indeed they know much about it in the first place. At the broad national level, the education of doctors is better conducted by doctors. In the first instance, this means through the Royal Colleges and the British Medical Association. The chiropody associations have a role to play in making appropriate information available. But the message will seem more credible if presented by doctors. It will look what it is, a more efficient way of distributing scarce health resources, and not an attempt at patient-rustling from rivals.

The DHSS could re-emphasise that aspect of the policy through health service administrators, In the long-term, better understanding of chiropody should be developed through the medical schools. But first priority must be to inform doctors already practising.

At district level, chiropodists must take the initiative in establishing firmer links with the different types of doctors to make sure that they know what chiropody can offer the various medical services. But at local level, contacts will have to go beyond education to negotiating new relationships – better cross referral systems, the better integration of both diagnosis and treatment.

That in turn implies an internal re-organisation of the chiropody service. If chiropody is to absorb the new referrals it negotiates, it must create the capacity to deal with them. Many suggestions to this end have been made by the authors, but it will inevitably be a long, slow process of change, which will have to be synchronised with the changing relationship between the doctors and chiropodists.

What is being suggested initially is modest and within the capacity of the chiropody service to absorb, if it achieves the efficiency gains described earlier. Each of the three types of doctors can be taken in order.

Surgeons

The suggested policy proposal here is for an immediate transfer to chiropodists of all in-grown toenail operations without further medical complications. Some uncertainty exists about the level of need for nail operations, because some of it may be concealed in waiting lists. But, even the chiropody services as presently organised could probably absorb this extra work.

Accident and emergency departments

The policy proposal here is for the integration of a chiropody service within hospital casualty departments. In practical terms, this would mean allocating the equivalent of one full-time chiropodist to this work. That is a more substantial commitment. In the research district, it would have meant giving 7% of staff to this work.

General practitioners

The initial aim is to increase the referrals of GP's existing foot patients. Since this involves the biggest potential change, it must be managed most carefully. Given the low level of detection by family doctors at present, large numbers of new patients would not be involved. But organising the referrals for prompt treatment would be a substantial administrative task and would have to be introduced gradually. The medium-term aims, however, include increasing general practitioners' detection rates, which leads naturally to increased referrals. In the long run, the aim would be to phase in various types of screening programmes.

Let us not pretend that chiropodists are volunteering to take on all this extra work just for the benefit of doctors or the NHS. It is hard for outsiders to realise the effect on morale of the present priority group system, which effectively means that many NHS chiropodists deal only with one type of patient, most of whose problems are incurable and who thus require repetitive treatment. Whilst the inefficiences in the way in which chiropodists deal with this problem have been pointed out, it must also be acknowledged how much monotony and boredom is structurally built into their work. Part of the solution to this problem is to create a more varied caseload for chiropodists.

Increasing the transfer of patients between doctors and chiropodists is thus a policy which benefits all parties and the NHS as a whole. Renegotiating professional roles and relationships is not a quick and easy task. But it can be done and it is worth doing.

30 Department of Health and Social Security: the case for action

The DHSS has great influence over many of the providers of foot health care, especially those working in the public sector. It is within the power of the DHSS to make policy changes in many areas of its jurisdiction.

First, in the area of training, the DHSS, by exerting influence on the relevant training bodies, could ensure that all relevant health workers, especially nurses and doctors, receive at least a basic grounding in the role that chiropodists play in the NHS, to provide a foundation for the process of matching the patients' needs to the appropriate skills. These two groups are particularly important as they not only constitute a large portion of hospital staff but also move out into the community; the former as district nurses, school nurses and health visitors and the latter into the School Medical Service, community physicians and general practice.

The training of most NHS professionals takes place in hospitals and thus students in the different professional groups have the chance to meet each other on wards or in out-patient clinics, despite their separate training. The majority of training schools for chiropodists are, however, within the further education (higher education) sector. This physical separation, along with the small number of students (1000 approximately) means that a doctor, and a nurse can complete their training without ever encountering a chiropodist (although it is unlikely that they will not have met a physiotherapist during the same period). The DHSS should, along with the CPSM, consider training chiropodists within hospitals, where the community in which they train more closely reflects that in which they will ultimately work.

The DHSS will, however, also need to face the problem of the small numbers of fully trained chiropodists, who will still be in short supply, even if the proportion of sub-chiropodial work which they now do were to be reduced. Whilst two new schools have been opened in the last three years, and others have increased their student intake, the number of chiropodists who passed the Society of Chiropodists' examinations and thus become eligible for state registration and National Health Service employment was only 276 in 1982. An expansion in the number of training places should continue if the profession is even to maintain its numbers, in view of the age distribution of existing NHS chiropodists. Simply increasing the supply of footcare assistants will not mean that we need fewer chiropodists; it will mean that the ones we have will be able to make some impression on the vast amount of unmet need. Training more chiropodists does, of course, mean spending more money (unlike many of the reforms in the footcare world suggested so far in this book).

The DHSS could also bring pressure to bear on the Department of Education and Science to make training grants for chiropody students mandatory rather than discretionary. It is currently possible for people to successfully apply for a chiropody training place and then find that they cannot obtain grants to allow them to take up training. Additionally, the DHSS could investigate the possibility of allowing health districts to employ successful applicants to training schools on a full-time salary, so that the student would work as a clerical officer/chiropodial appliance technician, etc, in the vacations during the three year course.

Regulation of sub-chiropodial personnel

Much emphasis has been placed on the need for sub-chiropodial personnel, in order to release chiropodists to do more highly skilled work for which they were trained. If this sub-chiropodial role is to be accepted by the profession, the DHSS will have to find a way to regulate these new personnel, so that they cannot set up as 'chiropodists'. It is suggested that some form of closure of the profession will prove the key to solving this problem. The effective blocking of the introduction of FCAs with their existing very limited job specification has already been demonstrated. If this role is to be extended, even to the type of work currently undertaken by some pedicurists (using scalpels to remove callosities), the DHSS will need the co-operation of state registered chiropodists in order to set up training courses. The training need not be as lengthy or detailed as that of a state registered chiropodist, as these 'sub-chiropodists' would have a specific area of practice, as do dental hygienists. But the *quid pro quo* of co-operation is likely to be closure.

The problem has exercised many people for many years, and a satisfactory conclusion has yet to be reached. The two main possibilities are: functional closure, and indicative closure. Functional closure would effectively restrict the provision of chiropody services to a small number of practitioners, thus restricting availability to the public. Indicative closure 'would give the means of distinguishing between registered and unregistered practitioners, but unlike functional closure it would not restrict the services available'. (DHSS Consultative Document, 1981). The DHSS will not be able to solve this problem alone, but, in the interest of the public, should not abandon the dialogue which it is currently having with the various chiropodial associations. In their turn, these associations must be prepared to compromise. But without the present writers taking any position on the ultimate outcome of such negotiations, the DHSS must resist the eternal temptation of democratic government to do nothing about a problem until it becomes a public crisis. It is the patients who suffer when needs are unmet.

An agreement on the issue of closure would also allow the DHSS, the CPSM and the various organisations for chiropodists to issue guidelines to registrants and members which would increase the use of 'sub-chiropodial' staff, by reassuring members of the profession that everyone's interests were being served. Dentists do not, after all, refuse to use dental hygienists, because they know that the hygienist is properly trained and subject to a code of conduct. Problems of insurance and supervision would then also be more easily resolved. With these issues out of the way, the establishment of training programmes would be a relatively easy and inexpensive task.

Organisational changes

The DHSS could then attempt to bring about further changes in the organisation of NHS chiropody services. A change in the pay structure, to provide a better career ladder and to improve conditions, would obviously help to increase the proportion of chiropodists who opt to work for the National Health Service, at present only 50%. However, this alone will not be enough. It may be more important to change the type of work undertaken. Variety of work is often quoted as a reason for going into private practice, although the study of chiropodists' views on scope of practice (see pages 156 to 159) would appear to show that those in the National Health Service feel they have more opportunity to use their more specialised skills.

The priority group system

This leads to the strongest recommendation to the DHSS – also the shortest and simplest: abolish the priority group system. The system was ill-thought out and has not worked in the way intended. One of the priority groups (pregnant mothers) has no special need for chiropody, two others (school children and handicapped people) receive very little chiropody treatment, and the group which receive most (elderly people) mistakes 'priority' for a 'right' and overloads the service with relatively minor problems, depriving others who need it more. As a rationing device for a scarce resource, the priority group system has worked poorly. For the foreseeable future, some apportioning mechanism for NHS chiropody must be devised even if all the other recommendations are implemented. But a better mechanism than the present one can certainly be developed.

The most logical alternative, and the one which the authors strongly recommend, is access in terms of chiropodial need. The privileged position of any social group would be eliminated and foot and medical conditions substituted as the criteria for treatment. There is an elementary justice in concentrating limited resources on those who need them most.

Although this would be a radical change in principle, it would be a moderate one in practice. Given the physiology of the foot and the long-term genesis of foot problems, many people with severe foot conditions are elderly. They would remain the service's largest patient group. The new criteria of access, however, would allow NHS chiropodists to concentrate their work with elderly people on those with serious foot conditions that genuinely need chiropodial skills. Those who needed only foot hygiene would then be served by the new sources of sub-chiropodial manpower discussed (see page 126), by expanding voluntary services, by other health workers, by the private sector, and, through better foot health education, by themselves. The NHS chiropody service would then have the capacity to treat other patients from the general population with serious foot conditions, whatever age they might be. In practice, the emphasis in provision would shift not so much from elderly to young people, but from minor to major problems, from palliative to curative care, from foot hygiene to genuine chiropody.

However, the only sensible long-term policy for chiropody is to shift emphasis from treatment to prevention. This is the aim in most areas of health policy. But it is even more necessary in chiropody than other areas. Because of skeletal deformities, many foot conditions are irreversible in advanced age. Cure is impossible, no matter what the intervention. The only option is frequent, repeated palliative treatments for the remainder of the patient's life. This is the most expensive possible way to provide treatment, more expensive by far over a period of years than even the most costly surgery.

Many changes in the chiropody service and elsewhere to transfer effort and resources towards prevention have been suggested. If a serious effort is ever to be made to prevent foot problems, something must be done about changing the shoes British people wear. That involves the shoe trade, both manufacturers and retailers, and increasingly, importers.

The voluntary effort of the trade will probably need to be supplemented by some form of outside pressure, at best from an educated public which refused to buy poor footwear, but, realistically, from government. This need not take the form of punitive legislation; more subtle and positive forms of inducement are available. But sooner or later the government must negotiate with the shoe trade to try to improve the nation's foot health. The DHSS will have to take the initiative. Such a course of action has already been embarked upon with the cigarette industry. The results have not been all that the health professions have wanted. But they are well in advance of anything done with the shoe trade about foot health. It is time the DHSS made a start.

However, health education is the most important part in any campaign for prevention. Here the DHSS could act as a catalyst for all those who have a role in such education. Many agencies will have to be involved: the next section will deal with this important subject.

32 Health education: key to prevention

In his primer, *A textbook of health education,* A. J. Dalzell-Ward, then Chief Medical Officer of the Health Education Council, devoted 192 words of his 328-page text to foot health. This is a fitting symbol of the state of foot health education in Britain today.

Knowledge of even the elementary pre-requisites of foot health is astonishingly low. Most elderly people in the present study did not understand, even when they had painful conditions, that shoes have an effect on feet. The lack of consciousness among the young is more comprehensible, since their foot problems usually do not give them pain. But when 70% of the children were wearing, unwittingly, inappropriate shoes, the level of ignorance among children about foot health has become excessive.

This is not a criticism of the Health Education Council. That undernourished agency faces unlimited responsibilities with a limited budget. If it gives foot health a lower priority than the authors would like, they can also appreciate that the problems the Council does confront are more life-threatening than the foot conditions they are concerned with in this book. Besides, the task we face in foot health education is well beyond the scope of any single agency, even a much expanded HEC. When ignorance is so deep and so widespread as it is about foot health, the process of correcting it requires education and educators on many fronts.

Such foot health education as exists at present is undertaken largely by two groups, chiropodists and the shoe trade. Both are largely ineffective. Chiropodists give advice on footwear and footcare during treatment sessions, but the profession is resigned to the fact that this makes little impression; either patients do not listen or they do not accept what they are told. It is a double failure. Not only is there no change in behaviour, but the patient's footwear may also limit the choice of treatments for the existing condition.

At best, the shoe trade's performance has always been patchy. Some manufacturers and retailers take the task seriously, others do not bother at all. The message about good shoes and good fitting for children has received some support from the media. Every autumn, at the beginning of the new school year, a flurry of articles advise parents how to choose their children's footwear. But when so many schoolchildren are wearing ill-fitting and/or badly designed shoes as this research discovered, the message is not getting through.

In many fields, health education is viewed as a peripheral or luxury supplement to the treatment services. But as has been stressed repeatedly throughout this book, the physiology of the foot means that many conditions cannot be cured if left until advanced age. Elderly patients already overwhelm the footcare services and their numbers are rising. Prevention is ultimately the only way out of the crisis in footcare. Central to prevention is foot health education.

The HEC cannot realistically be expected to do this job alone. As many resources as possible must be mobilised; in the footcare services themselves, in the shoe trade, among other health workers, and in other relevant organisations. But again, let the chiropodists begin by putting their own house in order, considering how to improve the educational work of the chiropody service.

The chiropodist's role

Commonly, chiropodists dispense their advice on a one-to-one basis, in connection with treatment, by means of rational argument. This is not the only way to educate people. In chiropody, as in tennis, if you are not winning, you must change your game. There is a formidable history of experiments with techniques of attitude change as guidance. In the health field, doctors and others concerned with weaning people off cigarettes, alcohol and drugs have tried many different methods. There may be a case for shifting from a positive to a negative strategy: from exhorting people to improve, towards scaring them with the consequences of inaction. The HEC had good results from its horrific campaign on seat belts, showing the scarred faces of people thrown through windscreens. Some of the foot conditions which chiropodists see daily would produce pictures at least as repugnant and frightening. The point is that chiropodists must reconsider their techniques of foot health education.

It must be acknowledged, however, that, regardless of technique, chiropodists face a serious structural limit on their educational work. The overwhelming bulk of their patients are elderly people with irremediable conditions. With them, even the most successful education will only be ameliorative rather than truly preventive. If chiropodists are ever to educate-for-prevention, they will have to communicate with a much wider range of the population than they do at present. In part, this entails treating a more varied mix of patients. But even more relevant in the educational context, is reaching out to non-patients, of all ages. This means taking foot health education out of the clinic into the community.

FCAs

Here footcare assistants could make a real difference, both in freeing chiropodists for more health education and in taking on some of this work themselves. FCAs themselves already give a modest amount of advice on a one-to-one basis, but there is a potential for substantial expansion of their educational role. Chiropody departments already receive many requests from community groups for basic information on footcare, more than they have time or staff to fulfil. With proper training, FCAs could take over and expand this work. Moving into the community involves more than a change of location; it is also part of a change in strategy, beyond retrospective individual advice to anticipatory collective education. Reaching large numbers of people before they become patients is the essence of any preventive health programme.

Foot Health Council

One positive form of chiropody transcending its traditional boundaries has been the creation of the Foot Health Council. It brings together a variety of interested groups, professional and commercial, national and local, which share a commitment to promoting foot health. Members include chiropodists, shoe manufacturers, shoe retailers, health education officers, teachers, doctors, public relations experts. The Council has promoted numerous activities since 1980. Its most ambitious venture so far has been the organisation of Britain's first 'Foot Health Week' in October 1983. The publication of this book was timed to coincide with that event. Both serve to emphasise how much needs to be done and how many are needed to do it.

The shoe trade

The most numerous potential foot health educators work in the shoe trade. And their influence comes to bear at a crucial point in the development of foot problems, at the moment of choosing shoes. But like chiropodists, they too must acknowledge that their past efforts have been insufficient and ineffective. In 1976, after prodding by the Office of Fair Trading (OFT) the major manufacturers and retailers agreed a 'voluntary' Code of Practice for Footwear. This is a positive development and has produced real improvements in shoe quality and the handling of complaints (*Which?* January 1980). But it does not deal seriously enough with the two areas central to foot health: design and fitting. Ideally, the improvement would come voluntarily. Another 'prod' from the government will probably be necessary, and this time it should involve the DHSS as well as the OFT. Potentially, the shoe trade is the largest foot health educator of all.

Too many designs are still being manufactured which are simply unhealthy for the foot. After decades of talking there is still no agreement on a uniform sizing system, and for adults there is little commitment to providing a fitting service. Here the situation is actually getting worse. For over a decade the government has been warning against any purchase of shoes by mail order, but this sector of the trade is growing. So are the self-service shops, but without serious efforts to compensate for the withdrawal of fitting advice by ensuring that customers can fit as well as buy for themselves. The trade has committed itself to improving staff training, but this training must put more emphasis on the provision of a fitting service for every customer.

Other health workers

Also very important are other health workers. All nurses who work in the community, district nurses, health visitors, and school nurses, could relatively easily and inexpensively incorporate foot health education into their work. The growing movement of community health workers has developed a large number of self-help programmes but has not as yet incorporated much information on foot health into these programmes. The authors' experiment in this area was not a great success, but it did not lessen the sense of potential in this work. Similarly, properly managed voluntary schemes could move beyond offering a simple nail cutting service and thus organise a substantial number of people for basic foot health education with vulnerable groups.

The education for change in this area, however, must come from chiropodists themselves. They must provide other health workers not only with the technical training and the back-up materials to undertake foot health education, but also with the motivation to make it a priority among many other commitments.

A latent potential for foot health education in other organisations could be realised. Schools could give it a more prominent place in their general health education. The consumer organisations could move beyond their traditional concern with shoes to campaign for better footcare services as well. In the longer term, employers' provision of preventive chiropody services could do a great deal to raise awareness of foot health.

And since one of the authors is a social scientist, something might be done to set that house in order too. Research by social scientists has been important in drawing attention to many social problems and in providing evidence to campaigning groups pressing for reform. But in the field of footcare, they have been conspicuously absent.

Interest in the economics of health has grown explosively in the last 20 years, but Culyer, Wiseman and Walker's extensive bibliography on the subject (see Appendix IV) contains nothing on foot health. The Office of Health Economics has never touched the subject. This is more than odd, since one of the principal justifications for giving elderly people priority access to chiropody is an economic one. Footcare is supposed to improve or maintain people's mobility, making them able to continue living in the community so that they are less likely to go into old people's homes, less demanding of home helps and other welfare supports. Everyone believes and asserts this to be true, but the economic case for chiropody has never been tested by economists.

Medical sociologists have concentrated their attention disproportionately on the élites of the field and have done virtually nothing with the literally and metaphorically pedestrian end of the health world.

In social policy, good studies of chiropody have been carried out as part of broader research on elderly and handicapped people, but heretofore only one book directly on the subject has been published (see Clarke, 1969). The increasing concern with the social problems of elderly people is improving matters, but as the limitations of the present research make obvious, there is still a great deal to be done.

There is even room for a psychology of footcare. Just before the present research was started, the district ran a poster contest for school children as a means of stimulating interest in foot health. The overwhelming bulk of entries concerned smelly feet. Now, bromidrosis is a serious problem for those who suffer from it, but is is such a relatively rare condition that, in a whole book on footcare, this is the first time it has been mentioned. But in the minds of school children, the dominant association with feet is smell. That is yet another symbol of the lack of foot health education in Britain today.

Training the trainers

Like most writing on health education, this section has been concerned with educating the general public – the final consumer of footwear and footcare. But at every stage, the groups nominated to do the education, themselves need education. We need to educate the providers of goods and services as well as the consumers. In fact, we need to educate them first. The state of foot health education is so poor, the task that needs to be done so great, that we need to start with the basics. Any serious strategy for foot health education in Britain must begin by training the trainers.

These proposals on health education were intentionally saved to the final section of the book, so that it might end with prevention. Health education is the key to any preventive programme and prevention is the central element in the strategy the authors have been developing for improving the foot health of Britain.

Many specific proposals for improving the **efficiency** of the principal footcare services have been made. Practical policies for an **expansion** of resources in chiropody have been suggested.

Inexpensive means of increasing screening among the young have been indicated, so that problems can be intercepted before they become incurable. But levels of need were discovered that would be beyond the capacity of even the most radically improved service to deal with. Need on that scale is what develops when a nation neglects foot health. If we continue abusing our feet the way we have until now, we will reproduce those levels of need generation after generation. For the majority of people, those needs will go unmet, just as they do today. The only realistic long term strategy for foot health is to educate people to take care of their feet, preventing problems from developing. The last word and the first priority must be prevention.

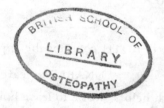

Appendix I: Questionnaire

THE CITY AND EAST LONDON
AREA HEALTH AUTHORITY (TEACHING)
DISTRICT CHIROPODY SERVICE

CLINIC   DATE   CHIROPODIST

NAME   DATE OF BIRTH   M/F

ADDRESS

GENERAL PRACTITIONER

MOBILITY: Please TICK, in BOTH columns the appropriate line.

ABLE to use bus alone   UNABLE to leave house at all

ABLE to use bus only with help   ABLE to leave house with help
or in wheelchair

UNABLE to use bus at all   ABLE to leave house alone

MEDICAL HISTORY: Please LIST all medical conditions, and all current medication, if any.

Diabetes mellitus	YES/NO
Rheumatoid arthritis	YES/NO
Neurological condition	YES/NO
Vascular condition	YES/NO
Other:	

ANY OTHER GENERAL INFORMATION RELEVANT: Please INDICATE below as appropriate and add any comments which would be of use to the next chiropodist.

Deaf	YES/NO	Able to remove shoes	YES/NO
Blind	YES/NO	Able to remove	
Partially sighted	YES/NO	socks/stockings	YES/NO
Use stick/frame	YES/NO		
In wheelchair	YES/NO		

What is the problem that has brought you to the chiropodist?

FOOTWEAR: Please INDICATE the type of footwear worn today.

ASK: Are those shoes the ones you usually wear?   YES/NO

If YES: ASK the following questions and RECORD as much detail as possible.

How much time do you spend in them?

What do you wear indoors?

If NO: ASK the following questions and RECORD as much detail as possible.

What type of shoe do you normally wear?

How much time do you spend in them?

What do you wear indoors?

ASK: Do you think that the type of shoes you wear has any effect on the condition of your feet? RECORD as much detail as possible.

ASK: Do you think a change of style might make a difference? RECORD as much detail as possible.

PREVIOUS FOOT HEALTH ACTIVITY

ASK: What made you apply for chiropody treatment?

ASK: How did you find out how to apply?

ASK: How have you been coping with your feet up to now?

ASK: Have you been cutting your own toenails?   YES/NO

    If YES, could patient be safely allowed to continue?   YES/NO

    If NO,

ASK: Has anyone been doing them for you?   YES/NO

    If YES, ASK: Who?

    Could they safely continue to do so?   YES/NO

ASK: Have you been attending a chiropodist or a pedicurist?   YES/NO

SPECIFY type by TICKING appropriate box	Chiropodist	Pedicurist
NHS		
PRIVATE		

CLINICAL EXAMINATION: Please TICK boxes as appropriate, and SPECIFY anatomical location for non-digital lesions in space provided.

SKELETAL CONDITIONS	RIGHT					Non Digital	LEFT					Non Digital
	1	2	3	4	5		1	2	3	4	5	
Hallux valgus												
Hallux rigidus/flexus												
Hammer/mallet/curly												
Over-riding toe												
Burrowing toe												
Syndactylism												
Amputations												
Pes cavus												
Pes planus												
Talipes (specify)												
Other skeletal conditions:												
Orthopaedic operations:												
Normal nails												
Onychogryphosis												
Onychauxis												
Onychocryptosis												
Involution												
Onychomycosis												
Digital corns												
Interdigital corns												
Digital callous												
Corns – not digital												
Callous – not digital												

CLINICAL EXAMINATION – continued

Please TICK boxes as appropriate, and SPECIFY anatomical location for non-digital conditions in the space provided.

	1	RIGHT 2	3	4	5	Non Digital	1	LEFT 2	3	4	5	Non Digital
Sepsis												
Ulceration												
Wounds												
Onychia												
Paronychia												
Maceration/ID fissures												
Fungal infection												
Hyperhidrosis												
Bromidrosis												
Anhidrosis												
Fissures (not ID)												
Verruca												
Naevi												
Scars												
Deep Tissue conditions:												

RECOMMENDED COURSE OF ACTION

Please INDICATE your recommendation for this patient below.

Your decision will need to be in two stages:

(i) the degree of urgency of need for treatment

(ii) the type of treatment plan.

MOST patients will have to be returned to a waiting list for treatment, only those in ACUTE need can be seen immediately. The rest will be sent for as soon as appointments are available.

Discharge completely

Annual check up only

Return to waiting list for treatment

Urgently in need of treatment

Having made this decision, would you now RECORD the treatment plan most suitable for this person when he/she can be accepted as a patient.

Advice appointment only

One treatment only, discharge

One treatment only, annual check-up

One treatment only, then footcare appointment

* Intensive treatment, discharge

* Intensive treatment, SOS appointments only

* Intensive treatment, foot care appointments

* Intensive treatment, long interval (20 wks+) appts. only

* Intensive treatment, then routine maintenance

** Routine maintenance

*give suggested number of treatments and interval
**give suggested interval

Appendix II: Caseloads for NHS chiropodists*

This basic norm has been agreed by the representatives of the following organisations:

The Association of Chief Chiropody Officers

The Health Service Chiropodists Association

The Hospital Chiropodists Group

The Institute of Chiropodists

The Society of Chiropodists

The norm applies to a full time chiropodist in the community service.

One chiropodist treats 16 patients per day (with clerical assistance, etc.).

5 days in a week = 80 per week
on a 6 weekly cycle = 480 patients
Rounded up, equals one chiropodist per 500 patients.

It is reasonable to assume that during the working week one day will be allocated for such things as schools, health education, appliance work, etc.

Therefore 4 days would be for the elderly group.

4 × 16   =   64 patients per week
on a 6 weekly cycle = 384 patients.

Therefore let us say that the ratio should be:
one chiropodist per 400 elderly patients.

Various surveys conducted have shown somewhat differing results; however, it is reasonable to assume that 50 per cent of elderly people will require chiropodial treatment (May Clarke suggested 90 per cent and Townsend and Wedderburn was nearer the 50 per cent mark).

Taking 50 per cent as a base-line, it would be reasonable to assume that the ratio should be –

one chiropodist per 800 elderly population.

Rounded up ratio of one chiropodist per 1,000 elderly population.

This norm does not take into account domiciliary and highly skilled and specialised treatments.

The Chiropodist, Vol. 33, August 1978, No. 8.

Appendix III: Sources of information

Clarks   *Tel:* (0458) 43131
Street
Somerset BA16 0YA
    Leaflets (small charge).

Children's Foot Health Register   *Tel:* (01) 739 3817
84/88 Great Eastern Street
London EC2 3ED
    Register of shops with trained staff for fitting
    and advice.

Disabled Living Foundation   *Tel:* (01) 602 2491
346 Kensington High Street
London W14 8NS
    Information services including books and
    demonstration kits on all aspects of footwear
    for problem feet.

Health Education Council   *Tel:* (01) 637 1881
78 New Oxford Street
London WC1A 1AH
    Leaflets.

Shoe and Allied Trades Research Association   *Tel:* (0536) 516318
Satra House
Rockingham Road
Kettering
Northants NN16 9JH
    Specialists and technical advice on footwear.
    Leaflets.

Society of Chiropodists   *Tel:* (01) 580 3227
8 Wimpole Street
London W1M 8BX

   Leaflets on all aspects of footcare.
   (small charge) including *Care of the feet for diabetics.*

Society of Shoe Fitters   *Tel:* (01) 242 7017
Carlisle House
8 Southampton Row
London WC18 4AW

   Advice on shoe fitting problems.

Start-rite Shoes Ltd.
Crome Road
Norwich NR3 4RD

   Leaflets.

William Timpson Ltd.
Southmoor Road
Wythenshawe
Manchester M23 9NU

   Leaflets (free).

Institute of Chiropodists
Ilford House
133-135 Oxford Street
London W1R 1TD

Tel: 01-439-8436

General Advice

Appendix IV: Bibliography

Age Concern. *Step on it!* Mitcham, Age Concern, 1976.

Association of Chief Chiropody Officers. *Survey of manpower resources in the NHS chiropody service.* 1980. ACCO, 3 New Road, Aston Clinton, Aylesbury HP22 5JD.

Black, J. A. and Coates, I. S. 'Silicones: their uses and development in chiropodial and prosthetic management'. *The Chiropodist,* 1981, vol. 36, No. 7, pp 237-251.

Bradshaw, J. 'Concepts of social need'. *New Society,* 1972, March, pp 640-643.

Chiropodists Board. *The Chiropodists Register,* London Chiropodists Board, 1980.

Clarke, M. *Trouble with feet.* London, G. Bell & Sons, 1969.

Culyer, A. J., Wiseman, J., and Walker, J. *A bibliography of health economics.* London, Martin Robertson, 1977.

Culyer, A. J. *Need and the National Health Service.* London, Martin Robertson, 1976.

Dalzell-Ward, A. J. *A textbook of health eduction.* London, Tavistock, 1975.

Davidson, P. 'A survey by a health care planning team in Solihull – chiropody'. *Health and Social Service Journal,* 1979, vol 89, No. 4655, pp 1044-1045.

Department of Health and Social Security, Welsh Office, Scottish Home and Health Department, Ministry of Health and Social (NI). *Proposals for statutory protection of professional title under the Professions Supplementary to Medicine Act 1960 and Closure of the Speech Therapy Profession.* London, DHSS, 1981.

Department of Health and Social Security. *Reorganisation of NHS and local government: operation and development of services, chiropody.* NHS Reorganisation Circular HRC (74) 33, 1974.

England, M. D. *Footwear for problem feet.* London, Disabled Living Foundation, 1973.

Harris, A., Cox, E., Smith, C. R. W. *The handicapped and impaired in Great Britain.* London, OPCS, 1971.

Hughes, J. *Footwear and footcare for adults,* London, Disabled Living Foundation, 1983.

Hughes, J. *Footwear and footcare for disabled children.* London, Disabled Living Foundation, 1982.

Jenkins, G. C. 'Footcare assistants'. *The Chiropodist,* 1977, vol. 32, pp 338-339.

Knight, R., and Warren, M. D. *Physically disabled people living at home: a study of numbers and needs.* London, HMSO, 1978.

Lewis-Clark, C. *The make-it-yourself shoe book.* London, Routledge and Kegan Paul, 1979.

National Consumer Council. *Bad fit, bad feet.* London, National Consumer Council, 1981.

Nevitt, D. A. Demand and need *in: Foundations of social administration,* ed. by H. Heisler. London, Macmillan, 1977.

New Zealand Government. *The chiropodists' regulations,* Wellington NZ, 1967.

Plank, D. and White, J. *Estimates of the need for the supply of chiropody services for the elderly in Greater London 1967-1991.* Pamphlet 16473. London, Greater London Council, 1974.

Savill, J. *Investigation into chiropody services in Camden.* Unpublished report, 1980.

Society of Chiropodists. 'Chiropodists and footcare assistants'. *The Chiropodist,* 1978, vol. 33, pp 97-99.

Society of Chiropodists. 'Case-loads'. *The Chiropodist,* 1978, vol. 33, pp 246-247.

Townsend, P. and Wedderburn, D. *The aged in the welfare state.* London, G. Bell and Sons, 1965.

Warren, M. D. *The Canterbury survey of handicapped people.* Canterbury, University of Kent at Canterbury, Health Services Research Unit, 1974.

Winkler, J. T., and Paley, J. 'Chiropodists and family practitioners: a study of attitudes and relationships'. *The Chiropodist,* 1983, vol. 38, No. 4, pp 118-123.

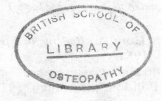

Index